# THE HIDDEN
# HEALTH CARE SYSTEM

An American Enterprise Institute Book

# THE HIDDEN
# HEALTH CARE SYSTEM
## Mediating Structures and Medicine

Lowell S. Levin
Ellen L. Idler

BALLINGER PUBLISHING COMPANY
Cambridge, Massachusetts
A Subsidiary of Harper & Row, Publishers, Inc.

This book was written under the auspices of a project on mediating structures sponsored by the American Enterprise Institute, Washington, D.C., and funded, in part, by the Division of Education Programs of the National Endowment for the Humanities.

International Standard Book Number: 0-88410-822-8

Library of Congress Catalog Card Number: 80-25060

Printed in the United States of America

**Library of Congress Cataloging in Publication Data**
Levin, Lowell S
  The hidden health care system.

  "Written under the auspices of a project on mediating structures sponsored by the American Enterprise Institute."
  Includes index.
  1. Social medicine—United States. 2. Social institutions—United States. 3. Family—Health and hygiene—United States. 4. Self-care, Health—United States. 5. Spiritual healing—United States. 6. Voluntary health agencies—United States. 7. Medical policy—United States. I. Idler, Ellen L., joint author. II. American Enterprise Institute for Public Policy Research. III. Title. IV. Title: Mediating structures and medicine.
  RA418.3.U6L48    362.1'0973    80-25060
  ISBN 0-88410-822-8

# DEDICATION

To Corinne and Philip

# CONTENTS

# FOREWORD

The term "mediating structures" may, in retrospect, be looked upon as a less than felicitous contribution to the English language. Still, whatever its lack of elegance, it refers to a phenomenon well known for a long time and designated in different terminologies by the social sciences—to wit, it refers to those institutions that stand between the individual in his private sphere and the large institutions of a modern society. In this location, mediating structures are, as it were, Janus-faced: on the one hand, they provide meaning and identity to personal life; on the other hand, they ensure that the large institutions, notably the state, do not lose their connection with personal meanings. Among these mediating structures, at least in America, a prominent role is played by the family, organized religion, voluntary associations, neighborhoods, and ethnic or racial subcultures.

The American Enterprise Institute project, "Mediating Structures and Public Policy," originated in a bias in favor of these institutions—not a romantic or reactionary bias, but one rooted in the conviction that these institutions are strategically important both for the well-being of individuals and for the vitality of a democratic order. The difference between social science and ideology is that, for the former, bias translates into hypotheses that can be empirically tested. The project as a whole was conceived as such a test. Specifically, it was designed to explore how public policy (especially that part of it commonly called the welfare state) in fact relates to mediating structures; beyond that, the project was to be an exercise in political imagination to reflect about how this relationship could be improved upon. This enterprise was perhaps not a "test" in the rigorous meaning of scientific method, but it sought to find empirical ways to assess the policy utility of the concept of mediating structures. To do this, the project was organized in five panels. Lowell Levin and Ellen Idler constituted the panel on health policy. Other panels dealt with criminal justice, education, housing, and welfare (especially as applied to children's services). Readers of the several publications will have to judge the success of the enterprise in its details. If the global hypothesis of the project was, stated quite simply, that the concept of mediating structures will be fruitful in thinking up new directions for the contemporary American welfare state, then I would assert confidently that the project has strengthened this hypothesis.

The book by Levin and Idler makes important contributions in at least four areas. First, and most directly, it contributes to the current discussion on health policy by drawing attention to a commonly neglected factor—the role of mediating structures. As far as I am acquainted with the current discussion, this contribution is pioneering; Levin's stature in the public health field and in the so-called self-care movement should give the book a fair hearing in those circles most concerned with the much needed reform of the health delivery system in this country and possibly abroad as well. This, in my opinion, does not exhaust the contributions of the book. Second, Levin and Idler make a contribution to the general discussion of what directions the modern welfare state should take. The specific case of health policy may then be taken as one instance suggesting new directions in other spheres of public policy. Third, their book demonstrates the applicability of sociological theory to some very practical concerns. Fourth, the book contains some highly intriguing "ethnographic" studies worth reading in themselves (namely, the "closer looks" at home childbirth, the Catholic charismatic movement, and rape crisis centers). In sum, this is a very rich book indeed, and readers with quite varied interests will find it rewarding.

My own interest (due to obvious professional deformation) is strongest in the second and third areas of contribution. But I would make an additional observation on the second area—the contribution made by Levin and Idler to the general discussion of public policy. They combine two qualities that are all too often separate—painstaking attention to empirical data and a radical vision of how empirical reality might be changed. I called this happy combination pedantic utopianism and argued that it was much needed in a situation crowded with technicians and prophets. Levin and Idler have contributed most refreshingly to the development of pedantic utopianism in the public policy field. It is not essential that one agree with all their positions to say this. I, for one, have some reservations (for instance, 20 million joggers strike me more as a manifestation of collective hypochondria than as a signal of self-empowerment). But Levin and Idler do not pretend to have all the answers. They have shown with great lucidity how certain problems can be looked at in a fresh way, they have indicated new avenues for empirical research, and they have produced a book that is a pleasure to read.

Peter L. Berger
Professor of Sociology
Boston College

# ACKNOWLEDGMENTS

The present book is one of several publications to emerge from the project "Mediating Structures and Public Policy" of the American Enterprise Institute. The project, which was partially funded by the National Endowment for the Humanities, ran for three years, 1977–79. Peter L. Berger and Richard John Neuhaus served as its co-directors. We would like to thank the AEI and especially the project's coordinator, Robert J. Pranger, for their generous support and for the freedom they have given us to pursue our research wherever it led.

Our assignment was to assemble as much information as we could on the role of mediating structures in health and to see what implications this knowledge might have for health policy. To this end, we would like to acknowledge the staff and resources of the libraries of Yale University, the New York Academy of Medicine Library, and the New York Public Library. A number of people have read and commented on earlier versions of the manuscript. Our revisions owe their considerable improvement to the patience and insights of Stanislav Kasl, Lee Hancock, Meredith McGuire, Mary Anderson, Eleanor Schuker, Susan Xenarios, and especially Alfred Katz. Of course, we accept all responsibility for those errors or oversights that remain. We would like to thank Patricia Moore for her cheerful research assistance and Margaret Gibbs and Vera Wardlaw for their skillful typing of the manuscript. We deeply acknowledge our debt to Peter Berger, who guided and inspired us through every stage of the project.

# INTRODUCTION

The time has come for a major conceptual shift in the health care policy debate, from viewing lay people as consumers of health care to seeing them as they really are: its primary providers. This book attempts to facilitate that shift by focusing on what may seem at first a fairly narrow topic: nonprofessional health care in American society. In spite of the pervasiveness and importance of the lay resource in health care, it has been largely ignored in the current debates over health policy. One must assume that it is overlooked because it is so thoroughly taken for granted, even (and especially) by health planners, professionals, and policy makers, the principle participants in the debates. Criticism of the professional health care system is ubiquitous; the system's numerous economic, social, political, and even medical flaws are well known. Although this work draws on the major criticisms of Ivan Illich,[1] Victor Fuchs,[2] Thomas McKeown,[3] and others, it will be primarily positive in tone, describing and advocating mediating structures, which we believe to be a powerful force in affecting and caring for the health of people who belong to them.

The first chapter examines the relation of mediating structures to individual health levels. The role of social support as an environmental factor affecting health is a topic of considerable current interest among leading social epidemiologists and medical sociologists, whose work is reviewed. With a few notable exceptions, very little research in this area has been undertaken with anything like the concept of mediating structures in mind, but research has moved more and more in this direction. The most recent work in this field does seem to indicate that there is a strong positive relationship between stable, supportive mediating structures and health and longevity.

The second chapter discusses the family and the health care activities it undertakes on its own behalf. The chapter begins by examining the literature on the family and self-provided health care in American history. Then it surveys current knowledge of the types, frequency, effectiveness, and safety of family self-care practices. Finally, it takes a closer look at the growing movement for childbirth in the home and some of the controversy surrounding it.

The subject of the third chapter is religious healing, with an emphasis on healing rituals and practices in mainstream Protestant and Catholic churches. Again there is some historical material and an attempt to survey the literature in the field today. This chapter concludes with a closer look at the increasing interest in healing among Catholic Charismatics.

The fourth chapter covers a range of groups found in most communities. These include the loosely organized network, which is mobilized in response to immediate needs; the currently prolific mutual aid group, a more formal structure of peers; and the new volunteer organization, especially telephone hotlines and peer-counseling services. The chapter closes with an account of the phenomenon of rape crisis centers, a new form of volunteer service organization.

The overall purpose of these three chapters is to lay to rest the assumption that "health care" in this society is synonymous with professional medical care. People perform a wide range of health care functions for themselves, some of which are quick and simple, some of which are long term and complex. Furthermore, there are historical and traditional bases for all of these activities.

The final chapter of the book explores the policy implications of mediating structures in health care. It assesses our present state of knowledge and indicates some directions in which future research might fruitfully be directed.

Mediating structures are not a panacea for all the problems of our health care system. We do not claim that for them. Indeed, it would be difficult to see how anyone could put such pluralistic groups to any unified use. In addition, there may well be liabilities associated with nonprofessional health care that can only be assessed by additional research. But it is our conviction, based on the research we have done, that it is in the interest of our society to allow mediating structures to operate freely in their own interest.

If our tone is positive, it is because we have experienced great pleasure in rediscovering a safe, personal, accessible, and inexpensive resource in health. We find the current groundswell of interest in health an encouraging sign of lay people's desires to increase their knowledge, skills, and responsibility in health, three of the elements of empowerment. It seems as if the existence of this resource can and does make a difference in people's lives and health.

It is currently fashionable in the health field to subscribe to increasingly holistic notions of individual health, by which is usually meant adding psychological, social, and even (to some) spiritual criteria to the definition. What we have discovered is that lay people have been including these criteria all along and acting in their own health interests in these broadly defined ways. Mediating structures are doubly vital to these definitions. First, they inform people's definitions of health in profound ways, through shared values and experiences. And second, they *are* what constitutes the social part of the definition. People include those who are most important to them in the way they think about the world. Any assessment of human health, then, either lay or professional, implicitly assesses the health and vitality of mediating structures.

We hope to show how mediating structures are a health resource at two levels. They constitute a most important aspect of the environment surrounding the individual, and they provide the great majority of all health care in this country. They constitute a valuable and vital social resource, which has been unappreciated because it has been taken for granted. This social resource is, however, too important to be overlooked and too essential to our social welfare not to be protected.

## REFERENCES

1.  Ivan Illich, *Medical Nemesis: The Expropriation of Health* (New York: Random House, 1976).
2.  Victor Fuchs, *Who Shall Live? Health Economics and Social Choice* (New York: Basic Books, 1974).
3.  Thomas McKeown, *The Role of Medicine: Dream, Mirage or Nemesis?* (London: Nuffield Provincial Hospitals Trust, 1976).

# 1 THE IMPACT OF MEDIATING STRUCTURES ON HEALTH AND ILLNESS

This book is about mediating structures, an unfamiliar name for the most familiar of social groups. The conception of these groups as mediators is one that could only come about in what we know as modern society. The structures themselves are not new. Indeed, those with which we will concern ourselves—the family, religious group, neighborhood and ethnic community, and voluntary association—are some of the oldest in human society. It is the fact that they mediate, that there is something for them to mediate *between*, that is peculiar to our present state of modernization.

The origin of this new function for these old institutions is to be found in the modern dichotomy between public and private life. Contemporary Western society is rather sharply divided between the megastructures that dominate the individual's public life as citizen, worker, economic consumer, and student and his or her private life as mother, friend, brother, husband. The megastructures, or large institutions, in our society are massive and powerful, exerting tremendous influence on the objective circumstances of our social situation, as well as on a large part of our consciousness of that situation. Most important among the megastructures, all of which are characterized by highly complex levels of bureaucracy or technology, is the modern state. But the vast bureaucracies of education and health care and the immense economic conglomerates of corporate business and organized labor are just as powerful and just as far removed from the individual's life. The intractable complexities of these institutions and their overwhelming influence, both subtle and overt, on the individual's private life can lead, not surprisingly, to a state of alienation or to a general feeling of powerlessness. These institutions are experienced as being "out there," unconnected to any sense of personal identity or meaning, capable of controlling but not of being controlled.

Typically, it is only in private life that the individual experiences a solid sense of identity and personal fulfillment. For most of us, it is only in our personal relationships that we can feel as if we would not be easily replaced. Yet the contemporary American's private life has become increasingly unstable. Identity demands that were once answered by one's work and the unique place this gave one in the community are increasingly placed on the small number of individuals who make up one's private sphere. The precariousness of this aspect of the social order, another condition peculiar to modern society, can lead to anomie, a lack of a strong sense of one's self and one's place in society. The break between public life and private life becomes sharper as one's public roles become more anonymous and as one's private life becomes more intense.

Mediating structures are located in, or better, across this widening chasm. They may be said to have two faces, one aspect turned toward the megastructures, the other toward the individual. Mediating structures can give stability to the private sphere, relieving it of some of its identity-providing responsibilities. As social structures they provide a variety of roles for the individual to fill and from which to construct a personal identity. They also constitute an opportunity for the individual to express freely a set of values in a concrete, socially objective way, giving a sense of their sharedness, as well as their effectiveness in influencing social action. Access to mediating structures can order the individual's own meaning system and integrate him in a community with a shared view of the world. In short, mediating structures alleviate anomie.

With respect to the megastructures, the mediating structure has a public face that represents an identifiable social group, which can be named (and even categorized) by the bureaucracy and which commands a certain amount of economic, political, or moral power.

Mediating structures provide a possibility for effective social action on a scale that is open to few single individuals in this society. They give one a handhold on a megastructure that would otherwise be both amorphous and intrusive. And, as a social expression of values, they may legitimate certain aspects of the megastructures and delegitimate others.

The concept of mediating structures, then, allows one to see some very old and familiar social institutions in a new light. These structures are to a large extent taken for granted by the people who compose them, which is just as it should be. They are real, immediate, and they can be counted on. The importance of belonging in such social groups has long been recognized, but it was Emile Durkheim who, at the beginning of this century, showed that the absence of such social groups in an individual's life could actually be a threat to that life.[1] Although Durkheim never used the term "mediating structures," the concept derives directly from his demonstration that suicide rates in modern societies are highest among those who are most isolated and who share the least in the collective life of their society. He showed social factors to be more important in determining suicide rates than any others, including physiology, insanity, race, heredity, and climate. Durkheim called the two types of suicide found most commonly in modern societies the egoistic and the anomic suicide. These names describe conditions in which individuals are insufficiently integrated in a social group or insufficiently regulated by a social group. Though Durkheim admits that the opposite cases can be just as bad, that too much social integration and too much regulation can also cause a person to commit suicide, these types are found much less frequently in individualistic and nontraditional modern societies. In modern societies like our own, then, membership in groups who share an identity and a tradition is found to be protective against suicide. Durkheim's thoughts on which groups should fill these roles are somewhat different from our own, but the way we see them working is the same.

Suicide may not be the only threat to life for which isolated individuals are at risk. Recent research in epidemiology, sociology, and medicine increasingly shows the relation of an individual's membership in social groups to a wide range of minor and serious, even fatal illnesses. Suicide may be only the most overt form of death from loneliness. In what follows we will attempt a chrono-logical review of some of this fascinating literature from the fields of social epidemiology and medical sociology. These groupings of the literature are admittedly arbitrary in some cases, especially when teams of investigators are made up from several disciplines. Nevertheless, certain clearly identifiable concepts have dominated the research in one discipline but not in the other. It has often been remarked that researchers in one field frequently seem to be completely unaware of the work on similar problems done by people in other disciplines. Though this may have been true of social epidemiology and medical sociology to a certain extent in the past, much of the research being done today in these fields is admirably well informed and indeed is often carried out by interdisciplinary teams.

## EPIDEMIOLOGICAL RESEARCH

Research in social epidemiology on the question of how mental and physical health is affected by an individual's membership in social groups can be traced back to the 1950s. Though the research reviewed here is highly relevant to the question of the role mediating structures may play in affecting the health of individuals, it should be cautioned that none of it has been done with the concept of mediating structures in mind. Yet these studies, many of which have used various measures of the very same groups we would identify as mediating structures, have been remarkably consistent in their results. The presence of close-knit social groups in an individual's life has repeatedly been shown to have a strong beneficial effect on physical and mental health. There is even evidence that the presence of such groups may lower mortality rates for their mem-bers. The significance of these findings should not be underestimated.

Investigations of how social groups affect human health and illness grew out of an earlier, more general finding that the social environ-ment seemed to be a significant factor in determining which seg-ments of a population were more likely to become ill. The best known of these studies were those done at the New York Hospital–Cornell Medical Center by Lawrence Hinkle, Harold Wolff, and others.[2] In their extensive studies of the health of more than 3,000 people in five relatively homogeneous population groups, they found that illness episodes, both minor and serious, were very unevenly distributed. During the two decades of study and for each of the groups studied, one-fourth of the individuals experienced approximately half of the illnesses that occurred in the group. The people who experienced the most illness had higher incidences of both minor and severe illnesses. Another major finding of these studies was that, within individual life spans, illness episodes are no more evenly distributed than they are within population groups.[3] Rather, illnesses of all levels of severity tend to "cluster" during certain periods of an individual's life, while other periods may be free of illness. The authors conclude that the key to understanding these distributions lies in differences in susceptibility that may obtain between groups within a population and between different periods in a single individual's life. Though the authors' explanations, that susceptibility varies with ability to cope with the environment and that illnesses occur when people perceive their lives to be "unsatisfying, threatening, overdemanding, and productive of conflict,"[4] may seem "soft" by today's standards, their studies do point up a clear association between bodily illness and conditions of the social environment.

The physiological basis for a relation between illness and the events and conditions of the social environment is to be found in the research on stress begun in the 1950s by Hans Selye.[5] Selye identified for the first time a patterned set of bodily responses to stress. The importance of this early work on stress was not the identification of any special characteristic of the social or physical environment as inherently *stressful*, but the establishment of a relationship between noxious stimuli in the environment (called stressors) and a pattern of bodily responses clearly recognized as a disease state. Moreover, the stress response was not linked to a single disease or even a group of diseases. Rather, these changes in the body's endocrine balance are currently thought to increase its susceptibility to the entire range of disease agents, thus invalidating earlier thinking that there was an identifiable set of "stress diseases."[6]

An immense amount of epidemiological research in the 1950s and 1960s investigating the effects of a stressful social environment on health was limited to measuring the incidence or prevalence of one or another disease entity thought to be related to stress. Many of these studies did produce significant and provocative results. One almost encyclopedic review of these early studies shows consistent relationships between the stressful social circumstances of unstable or nonexistent family life, and lack of social integration or ties to the community, and such diseases as tuberculosis, alcoholism, hypertension, heart disease, and cancer.[7] A few of these particularly interesting single-disease studies are worthy of note.

Thomas Holmes studied a representative sample of 200 institutionalized tuberculosis patients in a Seattle, Washington, sanitarium.[8] The proportions of 46 percent married, 21 percent divorced, widowed, or separated, and 33 percent single among his sample of patients differed significantly (at the 0.001 level) from the Seattle proportions of 65 percent, 9 percent, and 26 percent, respectively. The ratio of divorce to total marriages among his sample, 41.5 percent, was far greater than the contemporary national rate of 24 percent. In addition, he found that a large proportion of his sample, 74 percent, had lost the religious beliefs of the tradition in which they had been reared. He also noted that hospital medical records revealed that all the patients but one had "a striking and consistent history of poor health," including infectious diseases, accidents, operations, and behavior disorders.[9]

Another relevant study, this one of hypertension, was done among the Zulu of South Africa.[10] Blood pressure was measured for two groups of Zulu tribal people, one group that had remained on a reserve in a rural area, and another that had migrated to an urban area, Durban, South Africa. Certain stressful features were associated with both social environments: in the rural area there were problems associated with migratory labor and poverty, while in the city the Zulu experienced rapid acculturation in a modern, urban environment. Yet the study revealed that the mean blood pressures were higher for urban Zulu than for rural Zulu, at all ages and for both sexes. Scotch found that the differences in hypertension in the two communities could not be attributed to the presence or absence of stressful social conditions, which in fact could be found in both communities. Furthermore, the rapid social change experienced by the recent migrants to the city was not a sufficient explanation for the higher levels of hypertension found there, because it could not distinguish between the hypertensives and the normotensives within the urban group. Scotch argued that the actual stressfulness of a social situation for the individuals in it will depend on its social context. The crucial differences between hypertensives and nonhypertensives were in their abilities to adapt to rapidly changing conditions, and clearly some fared better than others. The ability to adapt, Scotch suggested, is modified by membership in certain social groups. For example, in the city, church membership is significantly associated with normal blood pressure among adult women. This study is just one of a body of research on social change and hypertension. One review of this literature concludes:

> People who are uprooted from stable communities, thrust into hostile, competitive urban environments in which their normal social institutions and reaction patterns make no sense, experience great elevations of blood pressure associated with this loss of control over the communal aspects of life. Adoption of social forms which more or less fit in the new environment (such as the nuclear family, fewer children) reduces blood pressure somewhat from this peak, but not nearly back to levels comparable to those in the stable rural social form.[11]

It may be worthwhile to mention another major study of the impact of social factors on the rate of coronary heart disease. This study took place in Roseto, Pennsylvania, a nearly pure ethnic community made up of first-, second-, and third-generation Italian-Americans.[12] The researchers reviewed the death certificates for the entire population of Roseto and four neighboring towns for the years 1955 to 1961. The results of a comparison were a much lower death rate from myocardial infarction in Roseto than in the other towns whose ethnic groups were mixed, including English, Welsh, and Pennsylvania-Germans as well as Italians. In fact the death rate from all causes was much lower in Roseto, especially among males between the ages of thirty-five and sixty-four and among males and females under fifty-five. The prevalence of myocardial infarction among men under fifty-five was also quite low. These results were somewhat surprising to the investigators, since the Rosetans also had a very high rate of obesity, the result of a diet in which 40 percent of the calories consumed were in the form of fat. A comparison of the coronary heart disease rates of the Rosetans with their male relatives who lived elsewhere also revealed the Rosetans' rates to be lower. Thus, neither hereditary factors, ethnic factors, nor dietary habits could explain their low rates. The researchers concluded that sociological factors were the most important and that it was the structure and the interaction of the community itself that made the difference. They found family relationships quite stable, close-knit, and mutually supportive, and the families themselves were supported by extensive networks of relatives. "The investigators were impressed by the way of life of the people of Roseto, particularly by their adaptability, their energy for work and fun, their hospitality, the stability of their families, and the cohesive quality of their community."[13]

These studies of the incidence or prevalence of some serious infectious and chronic diseases have been reviewed here at some length because, despite their great differences, some significant similarities can be found. Three of the studies reveal a relation between illness and what common sense would tell us are stressful situations: the broken homes of tuberculosis patients and the apartheid urban environment of hypertensive Zulu. But clearly there is more than a simple cause-and-effect relation at work here; not every urban Zulu became hypertensive, and not all divorced or widowed men in Seattle contracted tuberculosis. There must be some additional factors to make sense of these individual differences. The Hinkle and Wolff studies attempted to explain the individual differences in susceptibility apparent in their study in terms of differences in the way individuals perceived their lives; that those who experienced the largest amount of illness were those who perceived their lives as unsatisfying and overdemanding.[14] While this is certainly a worthwhile reminder that there is a subjective side to social reality and that all people do not perceive or respond to "objectively" similar situations in the same way, it does not go very far toward explaining why those differences in perception exist.

These studies, and many others like them, have repeatedly demonstrated this link between many different diseases and evidently stressful situations. As measures of tendencies in large groups of people, they have successfully shown significant connections. But most never even attempted to answer two far more difficult questions: What was it about these social situations that was stressful for people and why did some people in a situation get sick while others did not?

These two questions almost necessarily required a long period of time to be asked and thought about. They required a growth in empirical knowledge, in publicly available data about different communities, different social situations, and different diseases. By now the quantity of this research is enormous, and some very clear thinking has emerged. Perhaps more than anyone else, the late epidemiologist John Cassel is responsible for furthering this line of thought. In his 1975 address to the American Public Health Association, Cassel argued from both human and animal studies that there are two themes that underlie the research on social stress and disease. The first is a general characteristic of situations that explains why some are stressful, and the second suggests a reason why some people appear to be protected against the ill effects of stress. Cassel suggests that one important property of stressful situations may be that individuals are receiving inadequate or inappropriate feedback from their environment and thus are experiencing some disjuncture between their actions and their anticipated consequences. This would be the case for any individual who finds himself in a new and unfamiliar social environment, regardless of whether the individual himself moved or the situation around him changed. The recently migrated Zulu are certainly a good example of this property. The move from the tribal reserve to the urban community entails a radical change in the density of population and styles of work and living, not to mention a daily confrontation with the system of apartheid. The knowledge that an individual requires for getting along in these two environments is obviously very different, and the skills and years of experience acquired in the rural setting may be of little or no use in adapting to the demands of urban life. Some support for this interpretation is evidenced by the data, which showed that blood pressures were highest among the most recent migrants to the city and that they dropped off somewhat among longer term residents who had presumably had time to adjust to their situation.

The second of Cassel's themes concerns a set of processes more directly related to our concept of mediating structures. Cassel writes:

> These might be envisioned as the protective factors buffering or cushioning the individual from the physiologic or psychologic consequences of exposure to the stressor situation. It is suggested that the property common to these processes is the strength of the social supports provided by the primary groups of most importance to the individual.[15]

The groups that Cassel calls primary groups should not be taken as identical with our concept of mediating structures—this would be imputing too much for our own purposes. His last work on the subject mentioned family, work relationships, and religion as examples of groups that provide social support.[16] It would appear that the fit is close enough to be highly useful for a mediating structures approach. The way in which such social support actually protects the individual from the effects of stress has been the subject of much speculation and is still unclear; all that has really been established is that there is a relationship that seems protective of health.

Further illustration of these two points is provided by Cassel's own epidemiological studies in North Carolina. This series of studies began as an attempt to explain the health correlates of culture change in a rapidly urbanizing and industrializing part of our country.[17] They started with two hypotheses: (1) that the process of culture change in a community evolving rather rapidly from agricultural to industrial would be associated with changes in health status and (2) that the changes in health status would be most dramatic in those families "in which there is the least solidarity."[18] They defined culture as having two forms, one that provides the individual with a meaningful framework for living and for making sense out of life, and another that preserves social ties and the social structure they make up.

The first of these studies focused on industrialization as an aspect of culture change.[19] This research took place in a small industrial city in western North Carolina, which had a population of about 5,000 people. The town was one of many in that area experiencing rapid population growth as a result of industrialization. It had grown from a tiny mountain village of about 100 people to a town of 5,000 in just fifty years. The increase in population was the result of a decision by a large national corporation in the first decade of this century to locate a plant near the village and to draw its labor force from the local population. The people of the village and surrounding countryside were ethnically homogeneous, being mainly of British origins, and had lived in this rather isolated area for over a century. At the time of the study, workers at the plant could be classed in two groups, which the researchers called first-generation, and second-generation factory workers. The first group was made up of men whose fathers had been farmers. The second group had been the children of factory workers. The hypothesis to be tested was that the first group, for whom the factory situation was a new and quite different cultural context from the one in which they had been reared, would have higher indices of ill health than the second-generation workers, who had grown up in the homes of factory workers. Indeed, the results indicated that the first-generation workers had more total symptoms distributed in more different organ systems than the second group and a correspondingly higher absentee rate, which confirmed the original hypothesis.

The second of their studies focused on urbanization.[20] This somewhat later study encompassed the entire state of North Carolina and was designed to measure the effect of increasing urbanization on the rates of coronary heart disease. The authors expected that the rates of death from coronary heart disease would rise as the index of urbanism in each county rose. Death rates of all white middle-aged men in the state were examined for the years 1951–53 and 1959–61, and an index of urbanism based on the population of the largest city was constructed for each county. As anticipated, the rates of death from coronary heart disease (as well as from other types of heart disease) increased as the index of urbanism increased, and the latter index rose steadily over the period of the study. Most pronounced were the effects on rural residents, whose coronary heart disease death rates rose by 34 percent in the western part of the state and 37 percent in the eastern part. Urban residents of each county, on the other hand, who had presumably had time to adjust to their new cultural context, experienced a leveling off of their coronary heart disease death rates during the study.

These studies each attempt to isolate one factor in a changing cultural context and relate it to incidences of disease that cause, in one study, absenteeism and, in the other, death. Industrialization and urbanization are two facets of changing cultural conditions that rob individuals of the use of designs and values for living that may have suited their parents perfectly well. In both, changes occur from social structures based on kinship and extended family ties to those based on work roles where relationships are far less intimate. As individuals' interactions take place more and more between people who do not know each other well, if at all, responses and consequences of actions become harder to predict. This is the general characteristic of stressful social situations Cassel outlined.

The second theme, that of the role of primary social groups in protecting health, was foreseen originally by Cassel[21] but has only recently begun to be effectively researched by other epidemiologists. One of the first studies to attempt direct measurement of the effects of social support on health was that of Nuckolls, Cassel, and Kaplan, who studied the interaction of "psychosocial assets with life crisis and complications of pregnancy."[22] They argued that the connection between stressful situations and disease can be considered only in interaction with "supportive or protective elements." The study was done in North Carolina with 170 white women, married to military enlisted men, who were having their first babies. The measure of stressful social situations was the number and severity of life changes that these women experienced before and during their pregnancies. Measurement of "psychosocial assets" included information on marriage, family, and community relationships and feelings about self and the pregnancy. Pregnancies were judged to be "complicated" if they had any one of a list of nine characteristics, which included threatened or actual abortion, high blood pressure during labor, prolonged labor, or poor infant health. It was found that neither life changes nor psychosocial assets by themselves were significantly correlated with complications, which occurred in about 47 percent of the pregnancies. However, the results make much more sense when the independent variables are combined. Women who experienced the largest number of life changes before and during pregnancy had one-third fewer complications when their psychosocial asset scores were high than when they were low. On the other hand, in the absence of such life changes, psychosocial asset scores were not related to the outcome of pregnancy. In other words, the protective functions of these groups are only evident when there is something for them to be mobilized for or against.

This study of morbidity in a small population on the East Coast is supported in its findings of the importance of social support networks, by a West Coast study of mortality in a large population.[23] This research by Berkman and Syme followed up some earlier survey research done in 1965 in Alameda County, California.[24] They measured the impact of a range of social ties and networks on mortality from all causes. The types of social contacts the researchers measured in this study come closer than any others to our concept of mediating structures. The four sources of social contact they measured were (1) marriage, (2) contacts with close friends and relatives, (3) church membership, and (4) informal and formal group associations. Their results in each category indicated lower death rates among those who had such contacts than among those who did not. Given that these results measure not just illness but actual deaths and that the sources of social contact used are so similar to the concept of mediating structures, this study, more than any other, demonstrates the health- and even life-sustaining qualities of these four primary social groups. For each age and sex group in the population studied, mortality rates for the married were lower than for the nonmarried, whether single, separated, divorced, or widowed, and these differences were especially pronounced for men. In the second category, which measured both the numbers of close friends and relatives and how often they were seen, men and women at every age who reported few of these contacts had higher death rates. Third, those who belonged to a church or synagogue also had significantly lower death rates than those who did not, although these differences were not so great as in the first two categories, perhaps as a result of the differences between church membership and actual attendance, which was not measured. Finally, membership in all other groups also yielded differences in mortality rates in all age and sex groups but one, and these differences were especially pronounced for women. The authors of the study were aware that it is difficult to assess the direction of causality between social networks and sickness; that is, people may have few contacts because they are sick, or they may be sick because they have few contacts. They undertook to clarify this relation by controlling for health status at the start of the survey. This procedure demonstrated that at every level of health status, even among those who were already sick, those with the most social contacts had the lowest mortality rates. Furthermore, the existence of social networks was found to be positively related to good health practices, including not smoking cigarettes, drinking only moderately, eating regular breakfasts, not eating between meals, sleeping seven or eight hours a night, exercising, and maintaining normal weight, all of which have been demonstrated to contribute to physical health. Thus the encouragement of good health habits may be one of the ways social networks reduce mortality rates, but the authors caution that we are far from having a complete understanding of this process. The mechanisms by which social ties prevent disease and death might also be psychological processes that facilitate coping responses, or physiological changes in the body that increase susceptibility to disease in general. But regardless of what the actual mediating factors may be, the relation between social networks and physical health has been clearly demonstrated here.

The idea that social support could have a beneficial, protective effect on people's health is, as we have seen, not a new one in the field of epidemiology, though it has taken quite some time for epidemiologists to begin structuring their research to test this idea directly. In a recent review of the research on the subject, the authors note that most studies have formulated their notions of social support after the data were collected, to provide a satisfactory explanation of striking findings.[25] These authors outline an admirable and ambitious set of questions for future research, which could go a very long way toward explaining what it is about social support that is good for people's lives and health and also what implications these findings have for social and medical policy. More will be said about these issues later. For now, suffice it to say that the presently available research is so well done and suggestive that the importance of pushing these questions further cannot be denied. It should certainly be a goal of present policy to promote further research.

Thus far we have been looking at the slow but steady growth in awareness among epidemiologists of the importance of groups we have called mediating structures and their function of social support. Research on this topic in epidemiology has developed from an initial, rather vague awareness of the role of the social environment in affecting distributions of diseases in a population, through what must be called an obsession with the concept of stress and so-called stress-related diseases, to a growing focus on social relationships, or the lack of them, as the key factor in the social environment. One hopes that this admirable progress in research will continue.

## SOCIOLOGICAL RESEARCH

There has been an equally slow and steady growth of knowledge about the properties of these social groups within the discipline of medical sociology, which has come at these questions in a somewhat different way. Happily, social epidemiology and medical sociology have moved closer and closer to each other in their concepts and findings, though they have taken rather different paths to get there. Again, a caution is in order. The division we are making between social epidemiology and medical sociology is being used solely for heuristic purposes and should not be used to identify the authors of the foregoing or following studies as members of one or the other discipline. The operative distinction between the two categories is rather in their approach to and conceptualization of the relation between morbidity (and less often, mortality) patterns and social institutions and conditions. As we have seen, social epidemiological studies began with rather large-scale investigations of cultures or populations undergoing fairly rapid social change, or they studied individual groups within populations for whom social conditions were changing. The intermediate variable being studied was stress, and the dependent variable was either general morbidity or mortality or a measure of a specific disease, usually physical rather than mental, and characteristically chronic. However, research in social epidemiology has in recent years increasingly shifted its attention from the first of Cassel's two general themes to the second, generally confirming his prescience. That is, it seems fair to say that research interest has shifted from discovering the general properties of social conditions that are associated with disease to a study of the smaller scale social conditions that buffer or protect the individual against the first, that is, social networks and social support.

Medical sociology in this area, on the other hand, has had a much less clear chronological development with regard to these two themes, in both of which research has been going on for some time and continues to the present day. The first category of research has studied the effects of certain social events or conditions of social structure on illness within the population affected. There is a long history of research in sociology on the health effects of community crisis and unemployment, as well as the more general conditions of poverty and racial discrimination. The second category, which has developed simultaneously with the first, has been concerned with the conditions of personal life associated with illness. Until recently this research has focused on the health effects of stressful life events. Sociologists seem to have had a stronger interest in mental illness than epidemiologists, perhaps because the impact of the social environment is more obvious (though ultimately probably no more profound) than it is on physical health. As we shall see, research in this second category has recently turned from examining the negative health effects of conditions of personal life, ·which might be called the inverse of Cassel's second theme, to look at the positive health effects of social support and social integration. Clearly this second category provides the most information about mediating structures and health, and it is heartening to note that interest in research in this area is definitely on the increase.

### Large-Scale Social Factors

Let us briefly look at some of the social structural conditions social scientists have found to be associated with mental or physical illness. There is a significant body of research in sociology on the trauma of victims of disasters, especially those that occur in communities. Natural and man-made disasters are the most violent and extreme form of social change imaginable, often combining the highly stressful conditions of bereavement, personal injury, and destruction or complete loss of property. The subsequent impact of the unexpected loss of one's home, possessions, and even loved ones can be extremely traumatic and may be readily expressed as either mental or physical illness. One recent account of a devastating 1972 flood disaster in West Virginia movingly details the high toll illness took on the survivors.[26] The flood occurred when a makeshift dam made of waste from the local coal mine collapsed and allowed 132 million gallons of water mixed with solid waste to come crashing down on the small villages in the narrow valley below. The settlements nearest the dam were completely destroyed and carried downstream, and 132 people died violent deaths. Those who survived did so by running out of their homes and up the steep slopes on either side of the hollow, where they watched their homes being swept away and their neighbors being killed. A year and a half after the flood, psychiatric examinations of the survivors revealed that 93 percent were suffering from identifiable emotional disorders, including depression, anxiety, phobia, emotional lability, hypo-chondria, apathy, and insomnia.[27] Though it may seem somewhat inappropriate or unfair to classify these human reactions to a very real trauma as mental illness, the effects of continuous nightmares, sleeplessness, and vivid memories were recognized by the people themselves as debilitating.[28] Physical illnesses abounded as well. The most common complaint among the survivors was "bad nerves," which they tended to see as actual organic damage. Moreover, the connection between the destruction of their personal community and their current state of poor health was even verbalized by some of the victims. Erikson writes,

> The . . . speaker, a woman in her early thirties, is almost suggesting that the loss of neighborhood and community is related in some way to the loss of bodily function. And there may be something to that, for there is a sense in which separation from the familiar linkages of community is itself a form of illness. When one's communal surround disappears, and with it a feeling of belonging and identity, one tends to feel less intact personally; and one also tends to turn to illness as a way of explaining one's own dis-contents. This is why illness and disorder can become a way of life, a source of self-identification, a central fact of everyday existence.[29]

Erikson's work provides evidence of a strong link between the health of a community and the health of its members; damage inflicted on the former seems to manifest itself in the latter.

But not all social structural conditions that affect health do so through damage or radical change in the community. Some may affect health through their very constancy. The most obvious of these continuous social structural conditions is socioeconomic class. The effects of class on mental health and illness have been a subject of study for sociologists since the late 1930s, and this rela-tionship has repeatedly been shown to be a complex but important one. The classic New Haven study of the 1950s was designed to discover if there was a relationship between social class position and the manifestation and treatment of psychiatric disorders.[30] By studying the population of all individuals in New Haven in psy-chiatric treatment and comparing them with a systematic sample of all residents of the city, the authors were able to tell a good deal about the prevalence of treated mental illness, the types of diagnoses made, and the kind of psychiatric treatment administered. All these factors were found to be significantly related to differences in class position. These striking findings, however, are limited to the population that had found its way, for one reason or another, into the psychiatric care system.

A second classic study, done a few years later, attempted to measure the amount of psychological impairment in an untreated population.[31] The Midtown Manhattan study examined psychological dysfunction and social class in the population at large. Leo Srole and his colleagues found an inverse relation between economic status during childhood and psychological impairment of adults. This relation was particularly pronounced among the lowest and highest income groups.

It would seem safe to conclude, then, from these and many other studies that socioeconomic status in our society is an important aspect of social structure relevant to the mental health and illness of individuals. A recent comprehensive review of the literature on social class and mental illness notes that, in spite of the disputes over causal mechanisms and in spite of differences in family and community experiences within social classes, it is difficult not to be impressed with the consistency of results of so much research.[32] Of course, considerable refinement of concepts has occurred in the past twenty years. Two related topics that have been examined in some detail are the relationships of health and illness to work in modern society and to unemployment.

Two review articles concerned with the health effects of working in our society have concluded that research has produced contradictory and inconclusive results.[33] Some studies seem to show that people in higher status jobs have somewhat better mental health, but these are not very strong associations.[34] Furthermore, people in high-status occupations report more worry about their work and are consistently found to have higher blood pressure.[35]

But if the effects of occupation on health are too complex to be clearly predictable, the health effects of loss of work are not. One study undertaken in the late 1960s measured changes in health status, reported symptoms, and illness behavior among two groups of industrial workers whose plants closed down.[36] The authors chose to study the group for whom unemployment would presumably have the most serious consequences: married men between the ages of forty and fifty. The study was begun before the plants closed down but after the workers had been informed that the closings were imminent. The authors found that blood pressure was significantly higher during the periods of anticipation, unemployment, and the initial period of reemployment than it was after the adjustment to the new job had been made. Daily recording of symptoms revealed an elevation in complaints of common illnesses, colds, and flu, which was highest during the period of anticipation. The authors felt that these complaints did indicate some increase in the amount of real illness, although there was a disproportionate amount of medical care sought. These patterns were similar at both plants, one in an urban area and one in a rural area. However, the urban unemployed experienced significantly higher elevations in measures of cholesterol and illness symptoms even though their average period of unemployment was somewhat shorter than that of the rural workers.[37] The authors explained the urban-rural differences in terms of the importance of the role the factory played in the life of the community. In the urban area, the workers lived in many neighborhoods throughout the city. When the plant closed down, they lost the social support that came with daily contact with fellow workers. In the rural setting, on the other hand, the community itself was a source of social interaction and support, and the contacts with friends who had also been co-workers were not disrupted when the plant closed.[38]

Mental illness, too, has been shown to be related to economic change. One very large-scale study of mental hospitalization rates in the state of New York during the nineteenth and twentieth centuries shows them to be consistently inversely related to upturns and downturns in economic cycles.[39] Furthermore, it is precisely those segments of the population that lose the most in jobs, income, and social status that show increased mental hospitalization rates. The author concludes that instabilities in the national economy, as reflected in the employment rates of New York state, are the single most important source of changes in mental hospitalization rates and that this inverse relation has been basically stable for the last 127 years and does not appear to be declining in importance. "The major theoretical implication is that, despite our philosophic orientation, the destiny of the individual is to a great extent subject to large-scale changes in the social and economic structure that are in no way under his control."[40] The author even suggests that this greater vulnerability of the lower social classes to instabilities in the economy may be at the root of the often observed inverse relation between social class and mental disorder.

A final aspect of social structure that has been frequently studied is racial discrimination and its effects on health. Once again, however, it is difficult to isolate ethnicity from the effects of social class. One review of the literature in this area simply groups race and class as status-related sources of stress.[41] A later study of five ethnic groups in New York City argues that differences in ethnicity may account for up to 37 percent of the differences in mental hospitalization rates when the effects of social class are controlled.[42] This research shows the rates of mental hospitalization to be highest for blacks and lowest for Jews, with Puerto Ricans, Irish, and Italians, respectively, falling in between. When median income is held constant, these differences are reduced considerably but retain the same ranking. The authors argue that the high rates among blacks and Puerto Ricans are further exacerbated by differences in diagnosis and treatment rendered to members of these minority groups by mental health professionals.

These, then, are some of the large-scale social factors that have repeatedly been shown to be related to the mental and physical health of individuals. Natural or man-made disasters, poverty, unemployment, and racism all affect large groups of people in our society, some permanently, some temporarily. They are the kind of conditions that can make people feel powerless and unable to change their situation.

### Small-Scale Social Factors

Developing simultaneously with this research on social structural conditions has been a body of sociological research on the health effects of certain conditions of personal life. Like the large-scale conditions, research in this area has, at least until recently, tended to focus on the small-scale conditions that seemed to be associated with increased illness and death. Concepts in this field have moved through several distinct phases in the past twenty-five years and in this time have become more relevant to the concept of mediating structures. They have also moved closer to the language and methods of social epidemiology, so that the two sets of concepts are now virtually indistinguishable in this area.

Looking at this research chronologically, one would have to begin with the popular concept of stressful life events. The study of stressful life events and their effect on mental and physical health was originated by Thomas Holmes and others, whose early work on tuberculosis has been mentioned. Holmes and his co-workers believed that changes in people's lives that required them to make extensive adaptations or adjustments increased susceptibility to illness.[43] Some serious criticisms of this approach have been voiced, however, and it would seem that its popularity is now on the decline. In fact, some of the original investigators have themselves imposed a caution on the use of their instruments.[44]

The concept of stressful life events is only marginally related to our concept of mediating structures, just to the extent that such events concerned family members, which indeed some of them did. We have mentioned the concept because it illustrates extremely well how research in this field has progressed. The concept of stressful life events was a very good and useful way to proceed in investigating the ways in which the conditions of people's lives affect their health. Clearly these researchers were taking seriously what people said were important events in their lives. And given that these events were the ordinary events of human life that common sense would say were stressful, it is easy to see how promising the predictive value of the concept was. Some serious methodological problems have been raised,[45] however, and it would appear that emphasis in current research is shifting away from the concept.

Not all sociological research into the question of the health effects of conditions of personal life has been done under the rubric of stressful life events. Another major body of research, which in fact goes back further than the stressful events research, could be characterized as the social isolation/social integration concepts. Some of the earliest research in this area, which began in the 1930s, focused on the negative health effects of social isolation, schizophrenia in particular. One study was able to measure the rates of psychiatric hospitalization for schizophrenia in the different communities of a large city and compare them with several measures of social isolation.[46] The hypothesis, of course, was that the amount of social isolation would be greater in the communities with the higher rates of schizophrenia, and vice versa. In fact, the author found that residents of the highest rate schizophrenic communities knew significantly fewer of their neighbors by name, had lower estimates of the number of their close personal friends, and belonged to fewer lodges and fraternal organizations. This study was a truly sociological one in that it made no attempt to correlate social isolation with schizophrenia in individual cases, but in the Durkheimian tradition compared the characteristics of entire populations.

A review of some of the more case-specific early studies examined all those that had variations in family structure as a variable.[47] The authors conclude that parental deprivation, which included death, divorce, and separation, was found to be related to rates of a variety of psychiatric and physical diseases, including tuberculosis, ulcers, alcoholism, rheumatoid arthritis, psychosis, various unspecified psychosomatic diseases, and attempted suicide. They also review the studies of marital status and mortality rates, which have shown rather consistently that mortality rates are lower among the married than among the single and the previously married. Several studies show striking differences between these two groups with regard to death rates from influenza and pneumonia, syphilis, cirrhosis of the liver, tuberculosis, and accidents. Though the material reviewed is primarily clinical and epidemiological, rather than sociological, the authors do summarize the studies in terms of social isolation, which they define as "reduction of those social contacts and relationships which are of personal significance to the individual."[48]

One of the most interesting characteristics of this entire field of research has been its rather consistent one-sidedness in framing questions and hypotheses concerning these social factors and their relationship to levels of health and illness. That is to say, when one asks what the relation is between social isolation and illness, the unstated implication is that there is a corresponding relation between their opposites, namely, social integration and health. The language and hypotheses of sociological research have been thoroughly influenced in this regard by medicine and epidemiology, whose concerns are unquestionably disease oriented.[49] Epidemiology is, after all, the study of the distribution of disease in populations. There is no intrinsic reason, however, why sociologists should not be at least as concerned with factors that promote health and protect against disease as they are with those that may be associated with its cause.

Consequently, a number of sociologists have within the last few years begun to include values of social integration and social support in their analyses as factors in the prevention of illness and the protection of health. One of the first studies to incorporate this perspective was that of Jerome Myers, Jacob Lindenthal, and Max Pepper, who found the concept of social integration useful in explaining some data from their study of life events and psychiatric symptomatology that did not fit in the predicted patterns.[50] Their study of stressful life events and psychiatric distress revealed, in the majority of cases, a direct relation between the number of life events experienced in the previous year and the extent of psychological impairment. There were a number of people for whom this relation did not hold, however, that is, some people who had experienced few stressful life events reported many psychiatric symptoms, while some others who had few symptoms had experienced many stressful life events. These two groups were found to differ from the majority of people in the study in their level of social integration, which Myers and his colleagues defined as social class position, marital and family status, and employment satisfaction. Those in the group that reported few symptoms in spite of the presence of stressful experiences were of higher social status, married, and satisfied with their work; in other words, they were better integrated than the people with less eventful lives but more psychological impairment. The authors summarize their double-edged findings:

> People who have ready and meaningful access to others, feel integrated into the system, and are satisfied with their roles seem better able to cope with the impairment of life events . . . shared crises and mutual support appear to minimize intrapsychic disturbance. Conversely, unattached persons are more likely to be isolated and required to face problems on their own.[51]

The concept of social integration has taken a more structural turn in the work of some researchers in the area of social networks. The advantages of the social network concept lie in its quantifiability. A recent review of the epidemiology of mental illness and social class suggests that social networks are probably the most useful way to describe ties between the individual and the community.[52] They conclude that social networks play an important role in mediating the effects of social class on psychological disorder.

Another paper discussing these issues, however, argues that the concept of social support is the most focused and useful.[53] These authors review most of the social support literature and argue that the type of group that has been found to provide social support is the primary group. They point out that, like all groups, the primary group has both instrumental and expressive functions, and they identify the expressive functions as social support. Specific features of this expressive social support include (1) mutual caring and responsibility, (2) mutual identification, (3) emphasis on the individual's uniqueness, (4) face-to-face interaction, (5) intimacy, (6) close bonds, and (7) provision of security and affection. On the other hand, we would argue that effective social support cannot be simply expressive. Indeed, one could go even further and propose that social support by primary groups or mediating structures is powerful only to the extent that it is both expressive and instrumental. It makes no sense to say that affection from powerless groups can help individuals cope with problems.

We would like to suggest an alternative perspective on social support for future research, one that will include both expressive and instrumental aspects and that will reflect much more closely what we think is most important about mediating structures. First, the expressive functions of social support, described previously, can probably be safely condensed into two categories: (1) emotional expression and (2) identity provision and maintenance. Expressions of mutual caring and the intimacy that accompanies long-term relationships are most frequently thought of as occurring within the family but are found to a certain extent in all mediating structures. This expressive function basically describes only the face of the mediating structure that is turned toward the individual.

Families, however, are not strictly expressive when it comes to health and illness, as we argue in more detail in the next chapter. They also have an instrumental function, one more oriented to the larger society. This function, too, may be broken down into two categories: (1) its role in providing information and influencing judgment and perception and (2) facilitation of tasks. Mediating structures assist individuals not only in making decisions but also in carrying out the consequent action. They help interpret situations according to traditional, moral, religious, or other criteria and encourage individual action in harmony with the group's values and goals. Second, their instrumental functions include facilitating the performance of these tasks, which may be directed toward those within the group or those outside. The family and other mediating structures perform innumerable health-related tasks for themselves—

a description of these tasks is in fact one of the main goals of this book. But here we want to argue that *all* the tasks mediating structures perform are related to the health of the individuals who compose them. The competence of mediating structures to protect, support, and nurture the people within them seems, from the research we have been examining, to be rather directly related to measurable levels of mental and physical illness in individuals. While the specific health care functions of mediating structures are certainly important, they are not the only way in which mediating structures affect health.

It would seem that mediating structures do have a contribution to make to further research into the effects of social support on health. The concept of mediating structures can broaden the notion of social support beyond its expressive aspect to include its instrumental functions, the facilitation of decision making and tasks in all areas of life. The concept of mediating structures also has the aforementioned advantage of the social network concept: it is easily identifiable and quantifiable. It has another advantage derived from this; that is, it facilitates the move from policy to research. However belied by its name it may be, the concept is a common-sense one; everybody knows what families, churches, and neighborhood groups are. Research done with this concept in mind could have a direct and lasting effect on public policy in these areas, a subject dealt with in Chapter 5. At the moment it is enough to suggest that if research in the fields of social epidemiology and medical sociology continues as it has, we may be finding that the presence or absence of mediating structures in a person's life is the most powerful social determinant of health. The implications of this fact for policy are enormous, extending not just to health care policy but to all public policy that has an impact on families, churches, and neighborhood groups.

## THE LIMITS OF MODERN MEDICINE

Mediating structures, then, may be one more item on a growing list of social and environmental factors being found to have significant effects on our health. This new emphasis on moving beyond the single-factor theory of disease causation by investigating the health effects of the social and physical environment is associated with some important new research on the long-term effects of professional medical care. This question was first addressed by Thomas McKeown, whose historical research shows that the dramatic decline in mortality from infectious and noninfectious diseases during the eighteenth and nineteenth centuries must be primarily attributed to environmental influences, not to any medical discoveries of the time.[54] McKeown found that improvement in nutrition, in both the quality and quantity of food available, has been the greatest single influence on declining mortality rates. The other significant influences include sanitation and hygiene measures, which greatly reduced water- and food-borne diseases, and changes in reproductive practices leading to a decline in the birthrate. McKeown concludes from his study of the historical trends:

> The appraisal of influences on health in the past suggests that we owe the improvement, not to what happens when we are ill, but to the fact that we do not so often become ill; and we remain well, not because of specific measures such as vaccination and immunization, but because we enjoy a higher standard of nutrition and live in a healthier environment.[55]

McKeown's implication, that the health influences of medical therapy and immunization are small compared with the environmental and behavioral influences, is graphically illustrated in an article by McKinlay and McKinlay.[56] Their study of the decline in mortality in the United States since 1900 shows that medical measures have contributed little to the overall decline. In the cases of many of the major infectious diseases responsible for deaths in the nineteenth century, the decline in mortality (caused mainly by the factors noted) had begun long before medical science conquered the disease through prevention or therapy. They estimate that at most 3.5 percent of the total decline in mortality since 1900 can be attributed to medical measures introduced for infectious diseases.

Research such as that done by McKeown and by McKinlay and McKinlay constitutes a "modern heresy" that medical care is generally unrelated to improvements in the health of populations,[57] and it has jolted popular conceptions of the omnipotence of modern medicine. But economic research in the last decade has led to just the same conclusion. Grossman argues that the product "good health" is the result of many different kinds of investment, including diet, housing, exercise, and education, in addition to medical care, which is probably the least important of the five.[58] One study of the impact of increased medical services on the health status of individuals showed that increased access to and utilization of physician and hospital services produced no measurable health benefits.[59] The authors conclude that marginal increases in expenditures on medical services provide no improvements in health and in fact draw resources away from other programs that may have more beneficial effects. Another study finds that a 1 percent increase in the quantity of medical services in a population is associated with a reduction in mortality of about 0.1 percent.[60] It finds other environmental conditions, particularly income and education, much more highly associated with interstate differences in mortality rates. The effects of education on mortality are approximately double those of medical care and much less expensive to provide.

An enormous amount of money is being spent on health and medical care in the United States, and it is still increasing rapidly. Because of inflation, expansion of services, increases in accessibility, and the creation of new services, costs have increased threefold, from $39 billion (which was 5.9 percent of the gross national product) in 1965 to 192.4 billion (which was 9.1 percent of the gross national product) in 1978.[61] Yet health levels in the United States do not reflect improvement proportionate to increased expenditures. In 1975 the United States ranked eighth among twenty developed countries in life expectancy for women and fifteenth for men. Life expectancy for men born in the United States in 1975 was 68.7 years, about 3.5 years less than it is in Sweden. Average life expectancy has increased by twenty-four years since the beginning of this century, but for those who have reached sixty-five, it has increased by only three years. This indicates that the bulk of the improvement in life expectancy has come from improvements in infant and childhood mortality rates and that the average life span has not increased much. Infant mortality rates declined from 26.4 per 1,000 in 1955 to 15.1 per 1,000 in 1976. But in comparison with other developed countries, the U.S. rank has dropped from eighth to eighteenth.[62] This heavy concentration of our resources on providing medical services only underscores their marginal utility for improving health levels.

Economic resources are always limited, however wealthy the society. And the decisions about how they are to be distributed are always political ones. But currently, large-scale critiques of the way those resources are squandered in this country have come from such politically diverse members of the intellectual community as Ivan Illich and the late John Knowles.[63] Professional medical care is very expensive and getting more so. But its utility "at the margin," as economists say, is extremely small. We seem to be getting very little back for the enormous increases in costs we are paying.

### Iatrogenesis: Medically Produced Illness

Even worse than simply wasting our money is that medical services must not be considered completely benign. George Bernard Shaw wrote in 1911 that "the medical service of the community, as at present provided for, is a murderous absurdity."[64] "Iatrogenesis" is the word used to designate harm caused by medical practice, and, whether murderous or merely sickening, it is as old as medicine. But with the development of new diagnostic and therapeutic methods, some experts believe iatrogenesis to be increasing in geometrical progression.[65] Major disasters caused by medical practice include an outbreak of tuberculosis in Germany in 1930 caused by the administration of a vaccine containing live bacilli, polio caused by an incompletely inactivated vaccine in the United States in 1955, congenital defects in children of mothers who had taken the drug thalidomide during pregnancy in the early 1960s, and vaginal cancers among the daughters of women who were given diethylstilbestrol (DES) to prevent miscarriage.[66] A recent series of articles in the *New York Times* dealt with various manifestations of harmful medical practice: unnecessary surgery, unfit doctors, bad prescriptions, and unneeded and excessive X rays.[67] The articles estimate that 2.38 million unnecessary operations were performed in 1975, during which 11,900 people died; that 22 percent of the 6 billion doses of antibiotics consumed during 1975 were unnecessary, and that this 22 percent caused 10,000 fatal and near fatal reactions; and that 16,000 of the 320,000 licensed physicians in the United States are incompetent or unfit. A major study completed in 1976 by the American College of Surgeons and the American Surgical Association themselves found that nearly half the postoperative complications and 35 percent of the deaths studied were preventable.[68] The causes of 78 percent of these preventable incidents were found to be related to the surgeon.

Public consciousness of medical abuses and mistreatment has been an important cause of that distinctively American phenomenon: high-priced malpractice litigation. Approximately one doctor in ten is likely to be sued for malpractice in a year, but different specialties are sued with unequal frequency.[69] Surgeons are by far the most likely to be sued, and cardiac surgeons lead the list.

But the harm done to people by the medical profession is not at all restricted to the clinical iatrogenic effects of various mechanical and chemical interventions into the body, as Illich has so eloquently pointed out. The very diagnosis of illness, whether or not treatment is even undertaken, causes harm at other levels as well, which Illich has termed social and structural iatrogenesis.

An early, insightful article on the subject[70] outlines the norms governing the way physicians make decisions in diagnosis. Extrapolating from concepts statisticians use, type 1 and type 2 errors, Scheff argues that doctors are considerably more likely to judge a person ill who is really well (type 2 error) than the reverse, to dismiss a patient who is really ill. "'When in doubt, diagnose illness.'"[71] It is considered perfectly acceptable, "healthily conservative" even, to make repeated diagnostic tests and examinations on otherwise healthy people to rule out "suspected" illnesses. The logic of this rule requires a concept of disease as a "determinate" phenomenon that can only get worse if left untreated. It is also assumed that the diagnosis itself does no harm. But the diagnosis of illness entails a change in objective social status; at its most innocuous, the change can mean the simple and temporary taking on of the "sick role." At its most stigmatizing, it can become the beginning of a lifetime career of deviance. To move from the "unorganized" stage of illness, in which symptoms are experienced as subjective, unconnected, and preverbal, to an "organized" stage, in which symptoms become part of an overall disease pattern, complete with name, cause, and prognosis, also can entail massive changes in self-concept.[72] One begins to see oneself as a sick person. Scheff recounts numerous studies in which even symptom-free individuals, once diagnosed as having an illness, obligingly produced the appropriate symptoms.[73] It became a well-known fact during World War II that soldiers suffering from combat fatigue developed chronic psychological impairment if they were hospitalized for psychiatric treatment. Those who stayed with their unit recovered much more quickly.[74] The "decision rules" physicians appear to use, in which a clear preference is shown for diagnosing and treating illness that might not exist, rather than ignoring an illness that may exist, thus have important but frequently unrecognized consequences.

## Medicalization

In a way, this decision rule mechanism may be seen as the very basis of medicalization, the process in which medical practice increases its area of competence and utility by defining more human conditions as illness. If Scheff's two assumptions are applied to "problems" hitherto unrecognized as medical, they will be seen as (1) inevitably getting worse if left alone and (2) certainly not made worse by medical attention. Alcoholism, hyperactivity, and normal childbirth are good examples of phenomena only recently defined as medical. Whatever the mechanism, the increasing purview of medical practice is a historical reality.

An insightful article by Egon Bittner sketches the growth of what he calls "psychiatric influence," but it applies equally well to medicine as a whole.[75] He argues that psychiatric influence follows the decline first of religion and second of jurisprudence as "the background for thinking about collective life." Psychiatry in modern society functions

> not as a technical specialty, but as a fundamental approach to human life that functions cognitively at the same level as the conception of man made in the image of God and the conception of man as a rationally free member of a civic community.[76]

But where the two latter conceptions of man have long and rich histories, psychiatry is a new and highly modern way of thinking about the world and one's place in it. Bittner writes:

> Consider merely that in earlier times the sensibility and warrant of human conduct and of social ties were found in the criteria of morality and reason alone. It would have been absurd, or at least elliptical, to say that the choice of an occupation or a marital relationship was healthy.[77]

It was Irving Zola who originated the term medicalization and who, far more than Bittner, worries about its negative effects. Zola finds that the United States has a peculiar susceptibility to medical influence because of the strength of the values of activism, worldliness, and instrumentalism. He calls twentieth-century Western medicine "the great incorporator of knowledge."[78] Medical practice and research embody our society's most deeply held values and, tinged with humanism as they are, are thus "in a central position to be a codifier of the meaning of life in the 20th Century." They may indeed be "central" in the sense of being widely shared, but it would be a mistake to overestimate their power in individual lives. Medicine completely lacks the answers to the question of the meaning of living and dying that religion or even a set of ideological beliefs about history would provide. Individuals who lack firm beliefs about history or the hereafter might understandably be quite concerned about preserving their health and believing the promises of medicine. But medicine is only a plausible way of codifying the meaning of life *when it works*—that is, when it prevents death. When the meaning of life is reduced to the value of health, we can only lose our grip on things as we get older. Health is an inherently defeating thing to believe in.

Notwithstanding the strong beliefs in progress on which medical research is sustained, the intangible power of healing may be being lost as scientific knowledge is gained. Healing, an inherently social phenomenon based on the commonsense notion that health is more than just physical intactness, must be accompanied by human social interaction and support and can only be assisted by physical or chemical means. We will argue below that healing is based on shared values, symbols, and meaning systems. Unfortunately, these are exactly what is diminished as modern medicine becomes more scientific and removed from the experiences of everyday life.

## HEALING AND UNDERSTANDING ILLNESS

What we have been arguing for thus far are fundamentally social concepts of health and illness. From the literature examined in the first part of this chapter, it would seem that mediating structures play some role, possibly a very important one, in protecting the health of their members. The most current research defines this relationship in terms of social support but has yet to come up with a satisfactory way of explaining what this is and how it works. It is also clear, however, that social support is somewhat lacking in modern medical care and, even worse, that medicine may sometimes act to disable or discredit the social supports that people do have. In the last part of this chapter we want to look more closely at the makeup of social support in relation to illness and to show the precious, irreplaceable role that mediating structures play when people become sick.

To get at the ways in which mediating structures help people who are sick, it may be useful to look at an example of healing in a traditional society where these processes are more obvious. One set of cultural healing practices that has been intensively studied is that of the Navaho, so we will look at them in some detail.[79]

Traditional societies have specific and sometimes extensive stocks of knowledge about disease, what causes it, how it can be healed, and why certain individuals are afflicted and not others. Among the Navaho, knowledge about disease and healing is inseparable from knowledge about the Navahos' social and spiritual world. Indeed, the overall emphasis in Navaho religion is on divining the cause of and finding a cure for illness.[80]

The sick Navaho whose family remedies have been unsuccessful consults a tribal diagnostician, most commonly a "hand trembler," one of the three types of Navaho practitioners. For a small fee, the hand trembler goes into a trance and receives a diagnosis of and cause for the illness. For treatment the patient may go to either of the two types of Navaho healers, a curer or a singer. The curer is mainly consulted for minor illnesses or if no singer is available; he has fewer skills and charges much less than the singer.

It is the singer who is the best-known Navaho healer, the practitioner of chants and sand paintings. Becoming a singer is a difficult task. The efficacy of the healing ritual depends completely on its having been performed exactly right, and some ceremonials may last as long as nine days. Further, because the Navaho believe that every word of the various chants is sacred, none may be repeated out of the context of an actual healing. The difficulty of learning the chants has been likened to that of memorizing every line of the score from a Wagnerian opera only from hearing it performed.

The importance of the Navaho healing ritual, its healing potential, can only be seen in relation to the Navaho understanding of how disease is caused. It may be said that Navaho medicine is more holistically oriented than its Western counterpart. It minimizes the differences between mental and physical illness. Its guiding principle is that, through the proper use of ceremony and ritual, man can direct supernatural power toward two goals: removing or overcoming evil and restoring order. In the Navaho cosmology, these two amount to the same thing. Good is that which is under control; evil is that which is not.[81] Sickness is a manifestation of evil force entering a body from without and seeking to control it. Through the careful performance of ritual, the healer seeks to drive the evil from the body and from the community as well. Healing ceremonies invariably involve family members as participants; longer and more elaborate ceremonies for very sick people may involve much of the community. Their powerful effect is the re-affirmation of the essential solidarity of the community and its confidence in its relationship to the supernatural. Sickness, as the incursion into body and community of an uncontrolled evil force, is a threat to individual life and to the life of the community as well. Correctly performed ritual solidifies the community, giving it the strength to purge itself. Further, the suffering individual, rather than being isolated, rests at the center of a community that ritualistically washes him, feeds him, prays for him, sings for him, and paints beautiful sand paintings for him. What had been disordered in the community's relationship to the sick person is set right.

Navaho healing rituals provide an extensively studied example of a nearly complete juxtaposition of the religious and medical practices in a society and a set of beliefs about both that have not changed much in hundreds of years. When the efficacy of a ritual rests in its being learned and practiced *exactly* as it always has been, the encouragement for innovation is slight. These beliefs are thus practically unchanging and, even more important, must by definition be shared by all members of the community.

Such an overarching, comprehensive system of beliefs may be called a cosmology, or a symbolic universe.[82] It carries great authority because it integrates everything that the Navaho know about their world. The beliefs refer to a reality outside daily life, the supernatural, and indeed the rituals are not performed routinely, but only in the face of threat. In setting the most chaotic events in order, it allows the people present to *account* for every aspect of their lives. Thus the cosmology both represents the social order of which it is a part and maintains it.

Cosmologies are the product of past and present human activity in the world and as such are real in individual personal experience. Their ordering role in individual life includes making sense of personal biography and integrating disparate experiences. Illness certainly is one of the marginal situations that cosmologies must integrate. In ordering the individual's personal biography and current relationships to the institutional order, the cosmology provides the individual with a sense of himself as a member of a stable, historical social group.

Navaho society is one in which the cosmology is shared by all members of the society. In this case it is a specifically religious cosmology with a highly developed healing system inextricably linked with it. The Navaho cosmology derives its cogency, its inevitability, from its being the only imaginable way to think, to be, to speak, and to live. No group in our society, however, no matter how comprehensive and convincing its symbolic universe, can avoid knowing that there are other groups with other belief systems.

Of course, in a modern society not everyone shares the same cosmology, and there are even some cosmologies that are not religious at all. Some people may have a highly scientific cosmology that skirts the problem of the meaning of illness and death completely. Because religious beliefs so clearly influence the way people think about illness and death, the impact of other social factors on this knowledge may seem minimal. Research in sociology and anthropology, however, has demonstrated the existence of several ways in which human groups share beliefs about illness, whether or not they share religious beliefs. There may or may not be shared meanings on the conscious, verbal level in groups that lack a religious cosmology, but there are indeed shared meanings on a more subtle, preverbal level. This is a finding of great relevance for mediating structures, whose health-caring activities are, as we have seen, both expressive and instrumental.

Illness is an intense bodily, physical experience, however one may diagnose and treat it. The philosopher Gabriel Marcel once observed that human beings both *have* bodies and *are* bodies.[83]

This dual conception is a culturally variable thing, in that some people experience themselves as bodies more than others do. Any given individual may *be* her body more one day than the next or *have* her body during certain periods of her life. But there is one time, it would seem, that people would most especially *be* their bodies more than other times, and that is when they are sick. Of course these two conceptions of the self-body relationship are not mutually exclusive; no one can completely *have* her body or *be* her body if she is both human and conscious. Sickness, too, can take the form of a role that one plays (having an illness) or a subjective experience of pain or weakness (being sick).

It has been widely observed that there are distinct cross-cultural differences in the ways people express their pain and symptoms of illness. Zola's analysis of the presenting complaints of patients in a Boston hospital outpatient clinic revealed significant differences between ethnic groups with regard to the frequency of mental-psychological versus physical language about their ailments. The Irish and old-American groups were more likely to present diffused and unspecific physical complaints, while Italians and, to a greater extent Jews were more likely to couch their complaint in emotional language and speak about life problems, locating the illness in a social context.[84] Mark Zborowski's classic study of patients in a Veterans Administration hospital revealed that, with regard to language about pain, the Irish were the most stoic, Jews and Italians the most vocal. Of these two, Jews were more analytical, Italians more emotional.[85] These and other studies, in revealing the differences between expressions of illness by various social groups, also reveal a remarkable consistency of expression within the cultural and ethnic groups studied.

The roots of these common expressions lie in the universal but culturally informed human experience of the body. As the anthropologist Horacio Fabrega writes:

> The body must also be assumed to furnish the individual with a collection of rather elemental sensations that he draws on to give meaning and substance to his psychological and even social life. In this light, we must recall that illness in a fundamental sense reflects an alteration of the body—its shape, function, and feeling—and that for this reason, it also reflects and may trigger an alteration of the fundamental cognitive units that anchor the individual in his world. One is thus allowed to say that in changing the status and integrity of the body, the biological processes we have come to equate

with disease are associated with or mediate changes having wide-ranging implications, precisely because the body is composed of those fundamental verities that constitute for the individual the symbolic and/or cognitive units that in a phylogenetic and ontogenetic sense have created structure and order for him. Studies that probe basic meanings about the body thus promise to clarify not only what is universal and what is culturally variable about illness and/or disease, but also the central role that these intertwined notions have in man's perceived relationship to his ecosystem.[86]

Fabrega is suggesting that a very fundamental relationship exists among individuals, their bodies, and the social orders of which they are a part and that this relationship can be cast in high relief by the disturbance of disease.

Knowledge about one's body begins to be acquired in earliest infancy. The most important of early childhood socialization experiences concern bodily processes and their control. The knowledge that children acquire in their first few years of life, while they are learning to speak, eat, and eliminate in socially sanctioned ways, makes up the "fundamental cognitive units that anchor the individual in his world," to use Fabrega's language.

A recent study of family health behavior shows that families hold well-developed beliefs about health maintenance and that the family is the primary unit of health concern in our society.[87] The study also showed that the respondents were more likely to worry about another family member's health than their own, and this was especially true of parents for their children's health. But such early socialization experiences may differ in their use of language about the body and their social control system.[88] The knowledge that families teach their children about their bodies and the way they care for them communicate their set of values and way of seeing the world.

Some anthropologists have developed highly sophisticated schemes for explaining the strong and intimate bonds between the understandings of body and society. For example, the notion of boundaries applies equally well to bodily and social activity. In fact, Mary Douglas contends that, "the human body is always treated as an image of society."[89] Further:

The social body constrains the way the physical body is perceived. The physical experience of the body, always modified by the social categories through which it is known, sustains a particular view of society. There is a continual exchange of meanings between the two kinds of bodily experience so that each reinforces the categories of the other.[90]

She observes that the individual's bodily control will be most important in societies that emphasize culture above nature and those that are the most socially constrained. Moreover, social groups will tend toward a correspondence of activities and practices, particularly rituals, concerned with the boundaries of their body and the boundaries of their social group. Whether or not one accepts the structuralist basis of Douglas's argument, it seems fair to conclude that such linkages between the ways people conceive of their bodies and their social group exist, in whatever form and through whatever mechanisms.

Because these "fundamental cognitive units" are for the most part acquired during early childhood and maintained throughout one's life by one's closest associates, it may be said that these social meanings will be most highly shared among those to whom one is closest: one's family, community, or religious, social, and ethnic group. It is perhaps not too big a leap to say that the "alterations of the body" produced by illness will be perceived in common ways by these same groups.

Peter Manning and Fabrega, in an important paper, outline another sphere of socially shared meanings related to illness, in a way that neatly complements Douglas's view.[91] They begin by noting that Western social scientists studying other cultures have tended to ignore the social significance of the human body, by assuming it to be the universal equivalent of their own. But the modern Western view of the body, which they call "disembodiment," is largely a product of Western medicine and the germ theory of disease. Such a biologistic view of the body includes the following tenets: (1) organs and organ systems, and their specific functions, are identifiable; (2) the normal functioning of the body goes on pretty much the same for everyone unless disturbed by injury or illness; (3) people's sense experiences are universal; (4) disease and experience of disease do not vary from one culture to another; (5) boundaries between self and body and between self and other are obvious and shared; (6) death is the body's ceasing to function; and (7) bodies should be seen objectively.

On the other hand, traditional societies have a much more highly embodied sense of self. In their examination of the illness beliefs and medical systems of three coexisting groups in the Chiapas Highlands of Mexico, great variations in the sense of embodiment were found among the three groups. The first group, the Mayans, have a theory of disease similar to that of the Navaho, in that illness is first and foremost a social event, involving not the individual alone, but the individual's social group as a whole. Causation of disease is ultimately the action of the gods, as is the condition of one's spirit. Thus, just as the individual is viewed as inseparable from the social group, the self is firmly rooted in the body. One may say that the Mayans, like the Navaho, have a relatively undifferentiated senses of self: they *are* their bodies.

The second group, the Latino-Mestizos, tend to locate disease causation somewhat more firmly in the individual, through the concept of "illness propensity." Susceptibility to illness, however, is the result of changes in the personal environment that are more social than physical. The self is seen as continuous with the body, though it is to some extent differentiated, as it must inevitably become in a semiurban world. Illness is understood holistically, as the interrelation of body states and functions, interpersonal relationships, and emotions.

The third coexisting medical belief system is that of Western clinical medicine, whose biologistic bases with their thoroughly disembodied sense of self were outlined above.

Douglas and Manning and Fabrega have outlined two nicely balanced aspects of the ways in which groups of people and individuals go about the business of giving meaning to the experience of illness. All groups, even in modern societies, share a sense of their boundaries and a sense of embodiment. There will be great variation in these senses cross-culturally and even between groups within a society. But identifiable social groups will share such conceptions, and one is most likely to share such beliefs with the groups one is socialized by and into. These will very probably be mediating structures.

## MEDICINE, MEDIATING STRUCTURES, AND HEALING

Healing strategies engaged in by human beings in the face of illness are endlessly variable. But healing practices must be tightly linked to theories of disease causation and thus will vary along the lines indicated. The Navaho provide a good example of a nearly pure traditional type of healing system. Manning and Fabrega have outlined five principal characteristics of the Mayan and Mestizo healing systems that they studied, which would apply equally well to the Navaho and to other native healing systems that maintain a highly embodied sense of self.[92]

First, illness in the traditional healing system is conceived of in sociomoral and interpersonal terms. Rather than a set of role behaviors, it reflects concern with an altered state of human relationships. Body states alone do not constitute illness. Rather, illness encompasses a complex set of natural and supernatural events, states, feelings, and relationships.

Second, within this complex, the alterations in the state of the body of one individual rapidly radiate outward through the social group of which he is a part. Immediate family, kin, and neighbors in a broad network share the risks of and responsibility for the illness.

Third, because such societies have a wider kinship basis than that of the nuclear family in a modern society, the number of kin implicated in caring for the sick person and restoring her to health is much larger.

Fourth, the healing process in societies that have so broadly defined illness as a social state must be based on removing the social disturbances:

> Cognitive, affective, social, and moral disruptions in social relations (coded as illness) cannot be physically resolved by surgical intervention or by the use of drugs, nor can they be "psychologically" manipulated out of existence independently of altering the intrinsically relevant social patterns. Illness therefore cannot be privately resolved or cured, for it has social dimensions.[93]

Illness and healing are not conceivable in individuals isolated from their social group.

Finally, language about illness is the nonspecialized language of day-to-day relations. In fact, no separate words exist for bodily feelings apart from those used to describe interpersonal situations (shame, anger, disgust). The same words mean all these things. This is the source of a profound connectedness between self, body, and the social world, which we have described in the word "embodiment."

Healing in such a context depends on, and can take good advantage of, the power of the overarching set of symbols shared by all the people in the society. The cosmology maintains ultimate plausibility by virtue of there being no alternatives.

The importance of the social function of healing can only be seen with regard to the gravity of the situation in which it is shown. It is at precisely the situation of heightened anxiety about life and death that the healing potential of the individual's cosmology is called on. The imminent reality of death creates the most marginal situation of all, and "in situations of acute suffering, the need for meaning is as strong or even stronger than the need for happiness."[94] The reassertion of the strength of the society is a comforting thing. Identifying oneself as a connected part of a collectivity means that one can claim a very certain degree of immortality: the continued existence of the group. The individual who is able to locate her biography within the historical context of the group can make such a claim.

Unquestionably, religion has provided this integrating meaning longer and better than any other type of cosmology. But even if a social group holds no religious cosmology, it has been argued here that the most important social groups in an individual's life share a highly significant and relevant set of cognitive structures related to the body and its illnesses. Two symbol systems, one concerning the boundaries of body and society and the other concerning the relative sense of the embodiment of the self, are revealed in language, ritual, and beliefs about illness and are most fully shared with those with whom one is most intimate, in other words, one's mediating structures.

The consistency of language about the body, pain, and symptoms within identifiable social groups is plainly revealed in the Boston study mentioned previously.[95] Some ethnic/religious groups spoke openly about their illness and its psychological and social context. Others preferred to say little or spoke of the illness in strictly physical terms. Regardless of whether such patterns of interaction may directly affect healing, the importance of the pattern lies in its familiarity. Just as sharing the symbols is restorative of order and therefore comforting, so a confrontation with another symbol system may be disordering and threatening. Thus, even if a social group shares no explicitly religious explanations of suffering, its shared sense of the relations between self, body, and society provides a rich ground of symbols and meanings, which are highly relevant to the problem of illness.

The relationship of modern Western medicine to the phenomenon of healing that has been described is not a direct one, if indeed there is any relationship at all. Its major characteristics differ sharply from the characteristics of traditional systems elaborated above. The history of the development of Western medicine has been the history of the progressive disembodiment of the self. The body becomes endowed with an almost machinelike quality, complete with interchangeable parts. Body products and parts are all available to manipulation and retain no moral, sacred, personal, or unique meanings. As Manning and Fabrega write,

> *In primitive society the body of man is the paradigm for the derivation of the parts and meanings of other significant objects; in modern society, man has adopted the language of the machine to describe his body.* [emphasis in original] .[96]

Thus diagnosis and treatment are limited to the individual's symptoms, disease, and afflicted organ or organ system. Diagnosis is carried out by probing openings of the body and making openings where there are none, examining body products, and eliciting information from the patient. A successful diagnosis satisfactorily places the symptoms into a classification system shared by the practitioner and medical scientists.

Once diagnosis is complete, treatment is carried out through physical or chemical manipulation of body parts and processes, both inside and out. If some parts are found to be inadequate, they can be removed and replaced by others, either from other bodies, alive or dead, or made by machines from plastic and metal. The patient, as the sick individual in such a system is called, may experience a stripping away of identity as he or she becomes reduced to the limited totality of information on a chart. The disembodiment of self can even become a defensive reaction predicated on survival: the body, which has come so completely under the control of others, must be abandoned.

Western medicine also differs dramatically from traditional healing systems on the other theme we have developed: that of illness as a fundamentally social phenomenon. The body is treated as devoid of both self and social group. The causal link between disturbed social relations and bodily illness is ignored or passed over as too complex by medical scientists. Ironically, the discovery of social causes of illness has lately become a new, exciting field of research for Western social scientists.

The power of the Western medical system is great in displacing the indigenous healing systems in more traditional societies. But in a changing situation in which two or more systems for dealing with illness coexist, there is some evidence to suggest that people make reasoned decisions in choosing an alternative.[97] The individual's own beliefs about the cause of the illness appear to determine the resource from which help is sought; native healers are believed (correctly) to be better able to deal with supernaturally, morally, or socially caused illness, and the Western doctor is seen only in cases of naturally caused disease. Even in modern societies, such discriminations are made.[98] Among religious groups that practice faith healing, distinctions are made between impersonal, natural causes of illness and illness caused by sin, evil intent, or the breaking of religious taboos, and the services of the corresponding healer will be sought.

The phenomenon of medicalization in modern society was addressed earlier, but the link between medicalization and secularization should perhaps be stressed. Eliot Freidson notes the moralizing tendency of medicine and its progressive enlargement of its sphere of relevance.[99] Frequently professional and lay judgments about the existence and extent of illness differ; where the medical profession sees illness, the lay person may well see sin, crime, or eccentricity. The most likely area in which such differences may appear is that of psychiatry and mental health. The growth of the influence of psychiatry has been linked directly to the decline of the influence of religion and the law, in that order.[100] Psychoanalysis has been described as "a way of understanding the nature of man and an ordering of human experience,"[101] in other words, an attempt at a cosmology. Some people may even see psychotherapy as a kind of religious experience in which they discover their "true self."

But as close as modern medicine may come to taking the place of religion and even though psychotherapy may actually provide a functional equivalent of religious experience, neither of these can answer the questions human beings have about suffering, evil, death, and the meaning of their own lives. Certain writers have, however, viewed the doctor-patient relationship in just such ultimate terms.

Balint actually calls the doctor's work with patients the "apostolic function,"[102] by which he means the roles doctors play as teachers, comforters, father confessors, advisers, and so on. Frank acknowledges that psychiatric patients and their psychotherapists may not share value systems or "assumptive worlds," and so he argues that it is the business of psychotherapy to help patients make changes in their unhealthy assumptive worlds. Further, he finds that the best way to accomplish this change is in patients who feel dependent on the psychotherapist.[103]

Balint and Frank are physicians committed to clinical practice. Modern medical practice is largely incapable of providing personal or social meaning for an individual's illness experience. Clearly it carries no satisfying universal explanation for the existence of illness and suffering in the world. But neither do the practitioner and patient share many less ultimate values and symbols. Frequently their social contexts are made up of different classes, educational levels, and religious and political beliefs.[104] Chances are, unless the two are neighbors or friends, these matters would never even be discussed or known. The only possible cosmology that physician and patient could arguably share is that of modern science and technology, but this is only plausible when it successfully cures patients, which it certainly does not always do. In fact, it becomes needed most when it fails, in the face of death.

Because physicians and patients are no longer members of the same families and communities, whose members have always known each other, they also no longer share the self-body-society relationship outlined before.

> The vocabularies of medicine are not shared; specialized terms are applied to bodily parts and functions—the previous intimate connection between self, body, and interpersonal language and transactions is severed—for example, red corpuscles now become the locus of illness and the target for medical intervention. All these features tend to sharply etch the boundaries of the two worlds in which the patient and the physician live—social distance is marked in every word, gesture, and symbol employed. Money payment is but the final distinction that places the treatment experience in an impersonal, distant, neutral, objectified context.[105]

Modern physicians, then, share a very limited symbolic reality with their patients, which would in most cases not include religious understandings of suffering and death, common language or ideas about the embodiment of self, or notions about the boundaries of body and society. Such a situation, where healers and the sick are frequently strangers, not only to each other but to each other's social context, is unique to modern society and has emerged only in the last one hundred years.

In the past, Stanley Hauerwas argues, doctors in our society possessed considerably more moral authority.[106] They could be trusted with difficult ethical questions because they represented the community's wisdom about conditions necessary for a worthwhile life and a meaningful death. Doctor and patient were bound together in unspoken trust and mutual expectations. But this situation has changed radically. Today scientific medicine is symbolically empty. It has so removed itself from the normal social relations, language, and ideas of everyday life that it shares neither elementary cognitive systems nor overarching symbolic realities with anyone other than those who professionally share its reality.

The healing potential of mediating structures derives from these shared symbols, the meanings of which are acquired in early childhood and maintained throughout life by one's most intimate social relationships. People in mediating structures help each other interpret what is happening to them in terms of language and values that are understandable and meaningful to them. They attribute causes of illnesses that, as we shall see, are often surprisingly unmedical, and they make decisions about courses of action on the basis of these interpretations. Quite often these interpretations may be social, psychological, or religious in addition to or even instead of physical. Healing that is subjectively satisfying to the sick person cannot logically be accomplished without at least addressing itself to these other areas of the person's life.

To say that Western medical care does not attend to all the important aspects of a person's health and illness is not, however, to say that it could or should. Our society is a mobile, complex, and pluralistic one in which few people, if any, can expect to have doctors who are lifelong family friends. This role of providing caring, healing, and comfort can be performed only by mediating structures, and its healing effect should not be underestimated. It has been argued by some researchers in the field that the process by which social stress is converted to illness in individuals exists side by side with an opposite process by which social harmony produces healing and health. Manning and Fabrega write:

Psychosomatic notions of conversion have been pursued, it seems, primarily along the axis of how negative emotional tones are transformed or displaced on to bodily alterations without careful examination of the logically parallel process, found in our research, of elimination of pain and reconversion of harmony and well-being by the "infusion" of positive emotions and physical essences.[107]

It may be that mediating structures actually convert pain and tension in individuals into feelings of well-being and harmony that are measurable on some physical level. But in any case, the effects of the cognitive and emotional support of friends and relatives *feels* so good that people would probably continue to seek it, even if it were found to be bad for them. The healing social support given by mediating structures has perhaps been taken too much for granted. It is a unique and precious resource in health, which deserves recognition and protection.

## REFERENCES

1.  Emile Durkheim, *Suicide,* trans. John A. Spaulding and George Simpson (New York: Free Press, 1951).
2.  Lawrence Hinkle, Jr., and Harold G. Wolff, "Health and the Social Environment: Experimental Investigations," in Alexander Leighton, John Clausen, and Robert Wilson, eds., *Explorations in Social Psychiatry* (New York: Basic Books, 1957), pp. 105-37.
3.  Lawrence E. Hinkle, Jr., and Harold G. Wolff, "Ecologic Investigations of the Relationship between Illness, Life Experiences, and the Social Environment," *Annals of Internal Medicine* 49 (1958): 1373-88.
4.  Ibid., p. 1382.
5.  Hans Selye, *The Stress of Life* rev. ed., (New York: McGraw-Hill, 1976).
6.  John Cassel, "The Contribution of the Social Environment to Host Resistance, *American Journal of Epidemiology* 104 (1976): 107-123.
7.  Gerald Gordon et al., *Disease, the Individual, and Society* (New Haven, Conn.: College and University Press, 1968).
8.  Thomas H. Holmes, "Psychosocial and Psychophysiological Studies of Tuberculosis," in Robert Roessler and Normal Greenfield, eds., *Physiological Correlates of Psychological Disorder* (Madison, Wisc.: University of Wisconsin Press, 1962), pp. 239-56.
9.  Ibid., pp. 241-45.
10. Norman A. Scotch, "Sociocultural Factors in the Epidemiology of Zulu Hypertension," *American Journal of Public Health* 53 (1963): 1205-13.

11.  Joseph Eyer, "Hypertension as a Disease of Modern Society, *International Journal of Health Services* 5 (1975): 539–58.

12.  Edward N. Brandt et al., "Coronary Heart-Disease Among Italians and Non-Italians in Roseto, Pennsylvania, and in Nearby Communities," in Wilhelm Raab, ed., *Prevention of Ischemic Heart Disease: Principles and Practice* (Springfield, Ill.: Charles C. Thomas, 1966), pp. 217–25.

13.  Ibid., p. 224.

14.  Hinkle and Wolff, "Ecologic Investigations," pp. 1382–84.

15.  Cassel, "Contribution of the Social Environment" p. 113.

16.  Berton H. Kaplan, John C. Cassel, and Susan Gore, "Social Support and Health," *Medical Care* 15 (1977 Supplement): 47–58.

17.  John Cassel, Ralph Patrick, and David Jenkins, "Epidemiological Analysis of the Health Implications of Culture Change: A Conceptual Model," *Annals of the New York Academy of Sciences* 84 (1960): 938–49.

18.  Ibid., p. 944.

19.  John Cassel and Herman A. Tyroler, "Epidemiological Studies of Culture Change—I. Health Status and Recency of Industrialization," *Archives of Environmental Health* 3 (1961): 25–39.

20.  Herman A. Tyroler and John Cassel, "Health Consequences of Culture Change—II. The Effect of Urbanization on Coronary Heart Mortality in Rural Residents," *Journal of Chronic Disease* 17 (1964): 167–77.

21.  Cassel, Patrick, and Jenkins, "Epidemiological Analysis," p. 944.

22.  Katherine B. Nuckolls, John Cassel, and Berton H. Kaplan, "Psychosocial Assets, Life Crisis, and the Prognosis of Pregnancy," *American Journal of Epidemiology* 95 (1972): 431–41.

23.  Lisa F. Berkman and S. Leonard Syme, "Social Networks, Host Resistance and Mortality: A Nine-Year Follow-Up Study of Alameda County Residents," *American Journal of Epidemiology* 109 (1979): 186–204.

24.  N. Belloc and L. Breslow, "Relationship of Physical Health Status and Health Practices," *Preventive Medicine* (1972): 409–21.

25.  Kaplan, Cassel, and Gore, "Social Support and Health," p. 47.

26.  Kai T. Erikson, *Everything in Its Path: Destruction of Community in the Buffalo Creek Flood* (New York: Simon and Schuster, 1976).

27.  Ibid., p. 156.

28.  Ibid., p. 232.

29.  Ibid., p. 233.

30.  August B. Hollingshead and Fredrick C. Redlich, *Social Class and Mental Illness* (New York: John Wiley and Sons, 1958).

31.  Leo Srole et al., *Mental Health in the Metropolis: The Midtown Manhattan Study,* vol. 1 (New York: McGraw-Hill, 1962).

32.  Ramsay Liem and Joan Liem, "Social Class and Mental Illness Reconsidered: The Role of Economic Stress and Social Support," *Journal of Health and Social Behavior* 19 (1978): 139–56.

33.   Stanislav V. Kasl, "Work and Mental Health," in J. O'Toole, ed., *Work and the Quality of Life* (Cambridge, Mass.: MIT Press, 1974), pp. 171–96; Joseph Eyer, "Hypertension as a Disease of Modern Society," *International Journal of Health Services* 5 (1975): 539-58.
34.   Kasl, "Work and Mental Health," pp. 177–78.
35.   Eyer, "Hypertension," p. 548.
36,   Sidney Cobb and Stanislav Kasl, "Some Medical Aspects of Unemployment," *Industrial Gerontology* 12 (1972): 8-15.
37.   Stanislav V. Kasl, Susan Gore, and Sidney Cobb, "The Experience of Losing a Job: Reported Changes in Health, Symptoms, and Illness Behavior," *Psychosomatic Medicine* 37 (1975): 106–22.
38.   Susan Gore, "The Effect of Social Support in Moderating the Health Consequences of Unemployment," *Journal of Health and Social Behavior* 19 (1978): 157–65.
39.   M. Harvey Brenner, *Mental Illness and the Economy* (Cambridge, Mass.: Harvard University Press, 1973).
40.   Ibid., p. x.
41.   Barbara Dohrenwend and Bruce Dohrenwend, "Class and Race as Status-Related Sources of Stress," in Sol Levine and Norman Scotch, eds., *Social Stress* (Chicago: Aldine, 1970).
42.   Judith G. Rabkin and Elmer L. Struening, "Ethnicity, Social Class, and Mental Illness" (New York: Institute on Pluralism and Group Identity, 1976).
43.   Thomas Holmes and R.H. Rahe, "The Social Readjustment Rating Scale," *Journal of Psychosomatic Research* 11 (1967): 213-18.
44.   Minoru Masuda and Thomas Holmes, "Life Events: Perceptions and Frequencies," *Psychosomatic Medicine* 40 (1978): 236-61.
45.   George W. Brown, "Meaning, Measurement, and Stress of Life Events," in Barbara Dohrenwend and Bruce Dohrenwend, eds., *Stressful Life Events: Their Nature and Effects* (New York: John Wiley and Sons, 1974), pp. 217–43.
46.   E. Gartly Jaco, "The Social Isolation Hypothesis and Schizophrenia," *American Sociological Review* 19 (1954): 567-77.
47.   Edith Chen and Sidney Cobb, "Family Structure in Relation to Health and Disease; A Review of the Literature," *Journal of Chronic Disease* 12 (1960): 544-67.
48.   Ibid., p. 560.
49.   Ellen Idler, "Definitions of Health and Illness and Medical Sociology," *Social Science and Medicine* 13A (1979): 723-31.
50.   Jerome K. Myers, Jacob J. Lindenthal, and Max P. Pepper, "Life Events, Social Integration, and Psychiatric Symptomatology," *Journal of Health and Social Behavior* 16 (1975): 421-27.
51.   Ibid., p. 426.

52. Liem and Liem, "Social Class and Mental Illness Reconsidered," p. 151.

53. Alfred Dean and Nan Lin, "The Stress-Buffering Role of Social Support," *The Journal of Nervous and Mental Disease* 165 (1977): 403-17.

54. Thomas McKeown, *The Role of Medicine: Dream, Mirage or Nemesis?* (London: Nuffield Provincial Hospitals Trust, 1976).

55. Ibid., p. 94.

56. John B. McKinlay and Sonja M. McKinlay, "The Questionable Contribution of Medical Measures to the Decline of Mortality in the United States in the Twentieth Century," *Health and Society, The Milbank Memorial Fund Quarterly,* 55 (1977): 405-28.

57. Ibid., p. 405.

58. Michael Grossman, *The Demand for Health: A Theoretical and Empirical Investigation* (New York: National Bureau of Economic Research, 1972).

59. Lee Benham and Alexandra Benham, "The Impact of Incremental Medical Services on Health Status, 1963-1970," in Ronald Andersen, Joanna Dravits, and Odin W. Anderson, eds., *Equity in Health Services* (Cambridge, Mass.: Ballinger Publishing Company, 1976), pp. 217-28.

60. Richard Auster, Irving Leveson, and Deborah Sarachek, "The Production of Health, an Exploratory Study," in Victor Fuchs, ed., *Essays in the Economics of Health and Medical Care* (New York: National Bureau of Economic Research, 1972), pp. 135-58.

61. U.S. Bureau of the Census, *Statistical Abstract of the United States: 1979,* 100th ed. (Washington, D.C., 1979), p. 100.

62. United Nations, *Demographic Yearbook 1977* (New York: United Nations, 1978) pp. 151-57, 332-35.

63. Ivan Illich, *Medical Nemesis* (New York: Random House, 1976); John H. Knowles, ed., *Doing Better and Feeling Worse: Health in the United States* (New York: W.W. Norton, 1977).

64. George Bernard Shaw, *The Doctor's Dilemma,* preface (Baltimore: Penguin Books, 1974), p. 7.

65. Nikola Schipkowensky, *Psychotherapy versus Iatrogeny: A Confrontation for Physicians* (Detroit: Wayne State University Press, 1972); Robert H. Moser, ed., *Diseases of Medical Progress: A Study of Iatrogenic Disease* 3d ed., (Springfield, Ill.: Charles C. Thomas, 1969).

66. P.E. Sartwell, "Iatrogenic Disease: An Epidemiological Perspective," *International Journal of Health Services* 4 (1974): 89-93.

67. Boyce Rensberger, *New York Times,* January 26, 27, 28, 29, 30, 1976, p. 1 and continuing.

68. American College of Surgeons and American Surgical Association, *Surgery in the United States: A Summary Report of the Study of Surgi-*

*cal Services for the United States* (Chicago: American College of Surgeons, 1975).

69. "What's Ahead," *Medical Economics* (February 9, 1976): 278.

70. Thomas J. Scheff, "Decision Rules, Types of Error, and Their Consequences in Medical Diagnosis," *Behavioral Science* 8 (1963): 97-107.

71. Ibid., p. 99.

72. Michael Balint, *The Doctor, His Patient, and the Illness* (New York: International Universities Press, 1957), p. 18.

73. Scheff, "Decision Rules," pp. 102-3.

74. Ibid.

75. Egon Bittner, "The Structure of Psychiatric Influence," *Mental Hygiene* 52 (1968): 423-30.

76. Ibid., p. 427.

77. Ibid., p. 429.

78. Irving K. Zola, "Healthism and Disabling Medicalization," in Ivan Illich et al., eds., *Disabling Professions* (London: Marion Boyars, 1977), p. 48.

79. Clyde Kluckhohn and Dorothea Leighton, *The Navaho* (Cambridge, Mass.: Harvard University Press, 1947); Donald Sandner, *Navaho Symbols of Healing* (New York: Harcourt Brace Jovanovich, 1979).

80. A good summary of practices may be found in Bert Kaplan and Dale Johnson, "The Social Meaning of Navaho Psychopathology and Psychotherapy," in Ari Kiev, ed., *Magic, Faith, and Healing* (New York: Free Press, 1964), pp. 203-29.

81. Gladys Reichard, *Prayer: The Compulsive Word* (Seattle: University of Washington Press, 1944), p. 5.

82. Peter Berger and Thomas Luckmann, *The Social Construction of Reality* (Garden City, N.Y.: Anchor Books, 1967), pp. 95f.

83. Gabriel Marcel, *Mystery of Being,* vol. I (South Bend, Ind.: Gateway Editions, 1977).

84. Irving K. Zola, "Culture and Symptoms—An Analysis of Patients' Presenting Complaints," *American Sociological Review* 31 (1966): 615-30.

85. Mark Zborowski, "Cultural Components in Responses to Pain," in E. Gartly Jaco, ed., *Patients, Physicians, and Illness* (New York: Free Press, 1968), pp. 256-68.

86. Horacio Fabrega, *Disease and Social Behavior: An Interdisciplinary Perspective* (Cambridge, Mass.: MIT Press, 1974), pp. 12-13.

87. Lois Pratt, *Family Structure and Effective Health Behavior* (Boston: Houghton Mifflin, 1976).

88. Basil Bernstein, quoted in Mary Douglas, *Natural Symbols* (New York: Vintage Books, 1973), p. 50.

89. Ibid., p. 98.

90. Ibid., p. 93.

91. Peter K. Manning and Horacio Fabrega, "The Experience of Self and Body: Health and Illness in the Chiapas Highlands," in George Psathas, ed., *Phenomenological Sociology* (New York: John Wiley and Sons, 1973), pp. 251–301.

92. Manning and Fabrega, "Experience of Self and Body," pp. 273–75.

93. Ibid., p. 274.

94. Peter Berger, *The Sacred Canopy* (Garden City, N.Y.: Anchor Books, 1969), p. 27.

95. Zola, "Culture and Symptoms."

96. Manning and Fabrega, "Experience of Self and Body," p. 283.

97. Anthony C. Colson, "The Differential Use of Medical Resources in Developing Countries," *Journal of Health and Social Behavior,* 12 (1971): pp. 226–37.

98. E. Mansell Pattison, Nikolajs A. Lapins, and Hans A. Doerr, "Faith Healing," *The Journal of Nervous and Mental Disease* 157 (1973): 397–409.

99. Eliot Freidson, *Profession of Medicine* (New York: Dodd, Mead, 1975), pp. 252f.

100. Bittner, "Structure of Psychiatric Influence."

101. Peter Berger, "Towards a Sociological Understanding of Psychoanalysis," *Social Research* (1965): 26–41.

102. Balint, *Doctor, His Patient, and the Illness,* p. 216.

103. Jerome D. Frank, *Persuasion and Healing* (Baltimore: Johns Hopkins Press, 1961), pp. 31–34.

104. W. Timothy Anderson and David T. Helm, "The Physician-Patient Encounter: A Process of Reality Negotiation," in E. Gartly Jaco, ed., *Patients, Physicians, and Illness,* 3d ed. (New York: Free Press, 1979), pp. 259–71.

105. Manning and Fabrega, "Experience of Self and Body," p. 277.

106. Stanley Hauerwas, "Medicine as a Tragic Profession," in David H. Smith, ed., *No Rush to Judgment: Essays on Medical Ethics* (Bloomington, Ind.: Poynter Center, 1977), pp. 93–128.

107. Manning and Fabrega, "Experience of Self and Body," p. 270.

# 2 FAMILIES AND SELF–CARE

This chapter and the two that follow attempt to describe the hidden health care system in all its complexity. Our resources have been our own experiences and the available literature, both scientific and popular. We cannot claim to have been comprehensive; the field is both vast and incompletely explored. But we have tried to chart the terrain and to hone in on some selected topics where organized lay interest has preceded our own. As we shall see, the family, the church, and the community are significant sources, not only of social support vital to human health but also of health care.

The present chapter focuses on the family as the primary nonprofessional health care resource. It begins with a review of the family's health care functions in American history, a knowledge of which is essential for placing current debates in context. Second, contemporary self-care functions of families are inventoried and evaluated. The chapter ends with a closer look at one hitherto professionally controlled health activity that families are increasingly claiming as their own: childbirth in the home.

## THE FAMILY AND HEALTH CARE IN HISTORY

Although there are some difficulties in accounting for the health effects of the social support provided by mediating structures, evidence of direct care-giving activity is relatively more accessible. In this domain one can say with surety that mediating structures, particularly families, are the primary health care resource for most individuals in our society.

There is a popular misconception that health care is that activity performed by medical professionals. It is founded on the common confusion of the terms "health care" and "medical care." Popular confusion usually has its academic counterpart, and this case is no exception. The transfer-of-functions theory, first elaborated by early family sociologists in the 1920s and most recently embraced by Christopher Lasch, has been perhaps the most pervasive theme in American sociology of the family.[1] Broadly, this view of the recent history of the family is one of a progressive handing-over of previously familial functions to health, welfare, and educational professionals and institutions. Lasch provides an elaborate explanation of the intimate connections between this idea and theories of urbanization, in which the family was seen as an emotional refuge from an increasingly harsh competitive urban society. As its economic functions disappeared, the importance of its psychological and socialization functions became more obvious, at least to sociologists. According to Lasch, now these too are being taken away or given up. Without doubt, there have been some dramatic changes in family functioning in the past two centuries, just as earlier there were changes in its size and relative "definedness" with regard to the community. And it is certainly true that many educational and welfare functions have been taken over by the state. But to assert that any more than a small fraction of the caring for the health of people in modern society is done by medical professionals is to ignore a large amount of empirical data.

Talcott Parsons initially applied the transfer-of-functions argument to the care of illness.[2] He quite explicitly asserts that doctors and hospitals are "functionally alternative to" the family in the care of illness. Because of his conception of "the sick role" as both deviant and childlike, Parsons actually saw the family as inappropriate for the care of the sick. He preferred the legitimating authority and social control of professional medical institutions, finding that handling sickness outside the family served to discourage it in the first place. The point is not so much whether Parsons approved of such a state of things (it is obvious that he did) but that he took its existence for granted and started theorizing from that point:

We have given evidence which, we feel, indicates that the development of specialized professional health-care agencies, and *the consequent removal of much of the treatment of illness from the family,* is attributable to something more than the technological developments of modern medicine [emphasis added].[3]

Parsons's assumption needs a closer examination. It is undoubtedly true that there are more doctors, hospitals, medical procedures, and techniques than there were one hundred years ago. But to use this evidence of growth of the medical institution as a basis for concluding that the family's health care role has diminished is unwarranted and, neglects two well-documented social facts: the dramatic changes in disease patterns over the past three centuries and recent social changes in health practices.

Historically, of course, health caring for family members has always been an interest and function of families. Modern mortality rates show clearly that people get sick less severely and less often, and die later than they used to.[4] People in some parts of the country, and these were especially disease prone areas, once had no access whatever to professional medical help. On the frontier and in many rural areas, no doctors were available; so people learned to fend for themselves.[5] The inhospitable climate, lack of proper nutrition and clean drinking water, crude housing, and insufficient clothing all contributed to high death rates, especially among babies and children. Diseases that afflicted everyone included "remittent fevers," ague, malaria, "bilious fevers," cholera, typhoid, dysentery, consumption, pneumonia, "milk sickness," and smallpox, the vaccine for which was not available on the frontier. Medicines were made from wild plants, berries, barks, flowers, and roots, collected and prepared according to recipes shared by relatives and neighbors. Small communities usually had someone in them who was handy in caring for the sick, someone who was steeped in his or her own lore of cures, made up of observation, superstition, and home remedies, often of native American influences.

From the colonial period to the nineteenth century, urban areas of this country had similar disease outbreaks, and often their effects were exacerbated by large, dense populations. Epidemics of yellow fever and smallpox caused the nearly complete evacuations of Philadelphia in 1793 and Boston in 1721.[6] When people did become sick, they were cared for in their own homes, or in neighbors' if they had no immediate family. There was no alternative. When called at all, doctors came to where the sick person was.

The history of American medicine in the eighteenth and nineteenth centuries is one of a freewheeling climate, in which theories of disease causation competed for believers and the treatments that followed from the theories were as dissimilar as people's imaginations could make them. The so-called heroic practice of medicine constituted the mainstream of American medicine[7] (as, in a way, it does today). It was believed by the regular profession that the best therapy was that which produced the most rapid and dramatic changes in the patient's condition. Hence they used a small number of standard treatments for any ailment. These included bloodletting, drugs to purge the stomach and bowels, raising of blisters on the skin, tonics containing arsenic, and surgery without anesthesia. These dangerous and painful practices were surprisingly common, despite their unpleasantness and lack of therapeutic value.

But the practices of bleeding, purging, and blistering were hardly accepted by everyone. There were rival medical theories and systems with considerable followings that competed vigorously with one another. Several of these rival systems are of particular interest to a study of the history of family health care, because they promoted theories of disease causation and treatment that appealed to certain social groups, and they encouraged lay people to care for themselves.

The earliest significant leader of one of these movements was Samuel Thomson.[8] Thomson developed his own system of botanical remedies, based on the belief that the cause of all disease was cold. His book on the system, titled *New Guide to Health,* was not only a detailed guide to collecting and preparing herbs and nursing the sick with steam baths, emetics, teas, and tonics but also a direct attack on the regular medical profession. Thomson attacked bleeding, blistering, and the use of all poisons, as well as the general lack of education or experience in most members of the regular profession. But no theme in the book is more consistent than Thomson's criticism of physicians' high fees. No less than today, public displeasure with professional medicine centered on its high cost. Thomson's solution was for people "'to depend more upon themselves, and less upon the doctors,'"[9] by buying his book and teaching themselves. In addition to the book, Thomson set up Friendly Botanical Societies across the country, membership in which was granted with the purchase of the book. He employed agents in different towns to run the societies and sell the book; at one time there were 167 throughout the United States. Thomson started his movement in New England, but it had an even greater appeal in the Midwest and the South. With public opinion strongly in their favor, the Thomsonians actually succeeded in having medical licensing laws favoring the regular profession repealed in a number of states, including New York.

Thomson's movement was made up of the poor and others who had no access to doctors. Homeopathy, the other major challenge to heroic medicine, was quite the opposite: its physicians and patients were from the urban upper class.[10] Homeopathy was originated by Samuel Hahnemann, a German physician who became critical of regular medicine early in his career. He was particularly critical of what he considered the careless and basically ignorant use of drugs. Hahnemann reasoned that any drug, (such as cinchona bark, used to treat malaria), which causes the symptoms of an illness in a healthy person will cure the same illness in a sick person; *Similia similibus curantur,* "Like cures like." The more Hahnemann experimented with various dosages of drugs, the more he became convinced that the smaller doses of drugs produced "purer" symptoms and, in fact, that the smaller the dose, the more effective it was. He called these "infinitesimal medicines."

Thomson's movement and homeopathy, then, both opposed themselves to regular medicine, and both saw their own system as a safer as well as more effective alternative. But there was a sharp class difference between their adherents, and although both were widespread, homeopathy had a considerably stronger impact on the practice of regular medicine. The reason, of course, is that homeopathic physicians competed for the fees of the wealthiest clients of the regular physicians and successfully attracted many of them. Thomsonism was a challenge to regular medicine by the laity, and though it did eventually develop a certain professionalism of its own, it maintained a strong populist appeal. Homeopathy was originated and practiced by physicians; as such, it was a threat to the medical profession from within.[11]

Homeopathy did, however, have an element of lay practice, which contributed significantly to its popularity.[12] This was the "domestic kit," a case of carefully numbered infinitesimal medicines and a guide that prescribed treatments-by-number for most minor ill-nesses. These kits were clearly seen by the physicians who made them up as supplementary to professional care, not as an alterna-tive to it. The immense popularity of the kits is not difficult to understand. Instead of bleeding or purging, homeopathy offered pleasant-tasting pills that had no apparent side effects. The kits were especially popular with women, who found their children much more willing to "take their medicine." Homeopathic medicines were utterly safe, whether administered by physician or mother, and this was the ultimate strength of Hahnemann's system. The effectiveness of homeopathy rested on an as yet unrecognized character of disease: that it is largely self-limiting. Homeopathy simply allowed the body to heal itself, rather than violently disrupting the natural process as the heroic practices did.

Thomsonism and homeopathy were the two most important sects in nineteenth-century American medicine. They are important for our purposes because both contained strong elements of lay prac-tice and because they constituted the most organized opposition to the brutalities of heroic medical practice. But there was a consider-able amount of unorganized opposition as well, among people who simply refused to call a physician, preferring to treat their illnesses themselves with whatever resources were available. Chief among these resources were home medical handbooks, which began to be published in this country in the late eighteenth century.[13] The first of these books and one of the most popular was the Methodist John Wesley's book *Primitive Physick,* first published in London in 1747. Wesley combined his recommendations for the treatment of illness with sharp criticism of the medical profession. He believed that the contemporary medical practice of his day was simply a mystification of the common knowledge of herbal cures, which physicians used to raise their status and profits. He sought to return cures to their nat-ural simplicity: "Such a Medicine removes such a Pain."

Wesley's book of domestic medicine is somewhat unusual in hav-ing been written by a nonphysician, and this accounts for its critical stance. Most other domestic medical guides of the period were writ-ten by physicians who viewed their works as supplements to pro-fessional medical practice, to be used when no doctor was available or in cases of the mildest illnesses. William Buchan's *Domestic Medi-cine,* first published in America in 1795, placed much emphasis on prevention of disease through hygiene, wholesome diet, temperance, fresh air, and exercise. In addition, he prescribed a relatively moderate therapy whose role was "to assist nature." In 1826 Anthony Benezet wrote a handbook entitled *The Family Physician,* which was intended for use on the frontier, where few licensed physicians were available and disease outbreaks were serious, or on plantations where planters treated their slaves. These early handbooks, however explicitly intended for people without an available doctor, at least implicitly (if not explicitly) recognized the competence of families to deal with illness; after all, anyone could buy the book.[14]

In time, however, emphasis in the home medical handbooks shifted to the view that families should treat only the most minor illnesses themselves, that serious illness required the services of a physician. Thomas Cooper's 1824 *Treatise of Domestic Medicine* consisted of an alphabetical list of symptoms, diseases, and injuries, but frequently the only advice or information given was, "Send for a surgeon." Toward the end of the nineteenth century, authors of handbooks such as George M. Beard's *Our Home Physician* and Frederic M. Castle's *Wood's Household Practice of Medicine, Hygiene, and Surgery* turned more toward the task of educating the public to prevent disease and away from encouraging people to undertake their own treatment.

Besides reflecting various changes in the medical profession's ideology, these books had a significant impact of their own on the large numbers of people in the population who bought, shared, read, and followed them. And, as has been mentioned, serious illness was a frequent and common concern. That made these books valuable and reassuring. If a family had any books at all, they were likely to have a Bible and a domestic medical guide. It may well be that the growing interest in such books contributed to increasing dissatisfaction with heroic therapies. Given the state of medical knowledge in the first decades of the nineteenth century, it seems safe to say that home remedies could not have been less effective than medical therapy and may indeed have been safer by being more conservative.

The practice of health care in the home has been a topic of some interest for social historians of the nineteenth century, especially those interested in the changes in the roles of women. If women were not heroic medicine's especial victim, they were, as a group, its largest detractor.[15] It is also true that women, particularly, were concerned with matters of health and illness and became increasingly so as the century progressed. Growing interest in these issues must be interpreted in the light of the rapid and dramatic social change of the first half of the century and its impact on the family and women's roles.[16] The rapid growth of industrialization brought with it great changes in almost every aspect of the economic and social order. This was also a period of social unrest, and reform movements arose around a variety of issues including health and medical care, which we examine more closely in chapter 4. Women spearheaded and supported these movements.

The primary effect of industrialization on the family was the removal of work from the home. For working-class women, this meant leaving the home for work in the factory, wherever that might be located. Middle-class women found the economic importance of the home diminished and their own roles highly curtailed. Deprived of their economic importance, many women became involved in the "cult of domesticity," making the home into a small utopia into which family members could retreat from the upheaval and instability of the larger society. Thus there began in this period a rather rigid delineation of sex roles on the basis of work not characteristic of the colonial period, when families and homes had primarily economic functions. These rigid and mutually exclusive sex role behavior patterns did leave the nursing of sick family members to women, but this was not a burden to be borne by isolated individuals. Patterns of visiting and letter writing among middle-class women of the eighteenth and nineteenth centuries give evidence of the extensiveness and closeness of women's social networks.[17] Further, these networks turned around the most important events in the lives of women, providing considerable support, wisdom, companionship, and help. The subjects of these letters and the timing of the lengthy visits confirm the importance of the concerns of health and illness in this enclosed women's sphere. Frequent pregnancies, childbirth, nursing, weaning, illnesses, and deaths: these were the major events of women's lives in a time of relatively high birthrates, infant and maternal mortality rates, and frequent illness and death from infectious disease. The grief of sickness and death and the joy of birth were shared with sisters, mothers, cousins, and nieces, in an emotional world to which men were only peripheral.

It is no wonder, then, that women were so active in the health reform movement, given their primary responsibility for caring for the sick. Furthermore, the diminishing economic functions of the family and women's increasing opportunities for education necessitated alternative outlets for women's energies. Religious revivalism, moral reform, temperance, abolitionism, and women's rights were just some of the other, often overlapping social movements of the day.

Homeopathy, Thomsonism, the health reform movement, and other sectarian medical groups such as hydropathy, or water cure therapy, all had some impact on the practice of regular medicine. Taken together, they constituted a full-fledged revolt against the regular medical profession.

But it was advances in medical science that ultimately changed medical practice the most. The discovery of anesthesia and antiseptic methods allowed surgery to develop beyond its primitive, dangerous state. And the later developments in bacteriology led to the techniques of immunization and the understanding of the causes of infectious disease. These advances were not instantly accepted by any significant group of physicians, regular or otherwise; so it should not be thought that those who practiced regular medicine were any more naturally scientific than their counterparts. The new scientific medical profession was composed of the best educated regular, homeopathic, and other sectarian practitioners.[18] Changing medical education had its effect, though, and more and more young doctors learned to use microscopes and vaccinate for smallpox.

The subsequent developments of vaccines, sulfa drugs, and antibiotics in the first half of this century were among the greatest medical discoveries in history. Today there are effective vaccines or drug therapy for almost all the major infectious diseases that afflict this society, and mortality from the eleven major infectious diseases has declined from 40 percent of the total mortality in 1900 to just 6 percent in 1973.[19] As previously explained, medical measures alone do not account for this startling drop, the trend in infectious disease mortality rates having begun long before the medical measures were introduced. But the effectiveness of these measures cannot be underestimated either, and if they did not prevent many deaths, they did prevent or alleviate much infectious disease, and do so today.

It is over the acute, infectious diseases that modern medicine has established its hegemony and still finds itself set up to deal with, by prevention or cure. The relatively more frequent and severe episodes of acute illness of the seventeenth through the nineteenth centuries have given way to the two most frequent sources of sickness and death in this society, the ubiquitous minor illnesses and injuries of daily life: common colds and flu, indigestion, skin conditions, household accidents. The other major source of morbidity is chronic disease, which can vary in severity from hay fever to diabetes to cancer. These two types constitute by far the greatest proportion of disease in most people's lives, and they are precisely the diseases which are cared for, best and most often, by the family.

This shift in the kinds of disease most prevalent in our society and the spate of evidence of massive family self-care activity that we are about to examine are the two grounds on which we base our argument that the family has not given over its health care functions to the medical profession. Doctors and hospitals are not "functionally alternative" to the family, because they do completely different things. High-technology medical care of the gravely ill never did or could take place at home, and even its further expansion is not sufficient reason to argue that families have given up responsibility for the health and illness activities of everyday life.

The strength of Lasch's argument, more sophisticated than Parsons's, is his consideration of the process of medicalization in expanding the role of medical professionals. In bringing the medical-psychiatric perspective to bear on marriage and child rearing (in other words, families), the "helping professions" undermined the authority of the family at the same time that they emphasized its helplessness vis-à-vis the larger society.[20] They exacerbated just those conditions that were increasingly being identified as symptoms of mental illness: failure to cope, lack of ability to make decisions, avoiding responsibilities or commitments, and guilt. This was an effective way for the professions to make work for themselves. And of course the definitional expansion of illness to cover various types of social deviance—alcohol problems, sexual problems, overweight, juvenile delinquency—generated more work.

This expansion of the purview of professionals should not be seen as a strictly modern phenomenon, however. Modern feminist historians have documented the medicalization of women's condition in the second half of the nineteenth century[21] and medical advocacy of sexual surgery for a variety of nonmedical conditions.[22] Thus if medicalization as a process does create more actual sickness, it is nothing new.

What is new, and significant, is recent social change in the realm of health care and a new appreciation by lay people and even some professionals of the value of lay health activities. There is a significant effort under way in many nations to reappropriate health skills and to *re-redefine* conditions or events that had been redefined as medical by the medical profession.

The rest of this chapter surveys and evaluates the health activities of most families in self-care and of a small but growing number in home childbirth, two areas that are the subjects of increasing interest and controversy as families attempt to increase their own control and expertise in health and medical care.

## THE INDIVIDUAL AND THE FAMILY IN SELF-CARE

Like Molière's character who was surprised to learn that he was speaking prose, most people do not conceive of their ordinary, and sometimes extraordinary, life-sustaining activities as health activities, much less medical care procedures. Similarly, people are not accustomed to characterizing themselves as educators as they proceed to raise a family. And while many can easily see a given event as involving professionally identifiable tasks—just as completing an income tax form might be seen as an accounting task—few would acknowledge themselves as home economists in the daily business of household management.

Individual and family functions can, however, be parsed according to their respective disciplinary or professional reference. Such characterizations often serve purposes of research and policy development. We have seen the rationalization of child rearing as involving complex decisions and strategies that can influence the adult product. Indeed, the very decision to have a child[23] and under what circumstances has also been rationalized. Two new special interests of psychologists, educators, and pediatricians have been "bonding"[24] and "parenting".[25] The concept of role specialization in family function similarly has led to a perspective on the family as a technological environment, even an industrial environment, where the economic and social implications of work are accounted for.[26]

Evidence of this interest in the family is in sharp contrast to the conventional wisdom that the family, especially the nuclear family, is dead. Clearly, whatever has taken its place appears to be sufficiently powerful to present itself as a major target of blame for the alleged breakdown in American society. The perceived negative contribution of families to physical, mental, social, and demographic health precipitated much of the trend to professionalize the family. The tone of commentary on the family is often remonstrative and moralistic. Invidious comparisons of contemporary family life with earlier versions seem most effective as a release for frustrations associated with the sequelae of rapid social change. It is the reformist cant of professional interest in the family that has the potential to penetrate the organic integrity of family function. Cloaked in the apparent objectivity of science, seemingly free of self-interest, positive in their outlook (promising better results), and practical in their approach, reform strategies can easily be uncritically accepted.

To turn an old wheeze around, "Every silver lining has a cloud." The cloud in this situation is the latent potential for professionalizing the family and, in the specific case of health, medicalizing it. The raising to consciousness of the fact that life-coping behaviors have rational elements, both technical and conceptual, that can be improved is in itself potentially hazardous. Many indigenous practices have emerged from historical test and may depend for their effectiveness on an integrated, interacting set of values and beliefs. It may well be that their effective power lies in the family's commitment to them and to their symbolic contribution to family identity. The replacement of some indigenous practices by professional strategies might in such instances offer little or no technical advantage while eroding the integrity of the family's capacity for healing and caring.

Medicalizing family life functions makes such functions eligible for critique against the standard external criteria of medicine, the referent discipline. Affirmation and approval by external authorities is thus an added element in the family decision-making process. It is, in effect, a regulatory incursion into the private space of family life, the establishment of multiple miniprotocols of correct health procedures, which indicate the appropriate limits of lay health care as designated by professionals.[27] Family conformity and professional management predispose families to what Illich described as structural iatrogenesis, restriction of "the vital autonomy of people by undermining their competence in growing up, caring for each other"[28] When individuals and families are characterized as an element in the health care system as defined by the industrial values of that *system*, the portent of cooptation exists. Questions of a distinctly managerial bias then dominate research and development in family health: How can we (professionals) encourage more appropriate health behavior in families? How can we increase effective use of professional care services? How can we achieve better communication and coordination between patients and the health care system? How do we best share responsibility in decision making with clients? What is the approach to a partnership in health care? The seductive innocence of these queries masks an underlying assumption that establishes the professional care resource as the dominant health resource and casts the lay resource as residual, peripheral, and supplementary—except, of course, as a resource for disease prevention and health promotion, areas of little interest to the medical care system until recently.

What we must have is a professionally unbiased perspective on the family in modern society, its health role, and the relation of family health to external conditions and systems of disease causation, prevention, and cure. This can help thinking about ways of nurturing this social resource in health without manipulating the family toward the needs and goals of the industrial health care system. Unfortunately, no such unbiased perspective on the family, much less its health functions, exists. We are left with fragments of empirical data from studies whose variations in design, populations, and definitions make generalization hazardous. We are able at best to organize a multidisciplinary picture of family and individual health care rather than the ideal of a *multidimensional* picture free of professional distortion.

We shall undertake this mapping of individual and family health care functions by using the classical categories of health promotion behavior, disease prevention behavior, minor illness and injury care, and chronic illness management behavior. To these we shall add family behavior related to seeking and using extended-family and extrafamily helping resources, including both nonprofessional and professional resources, and individual and family behavior in control of iatrogenic effects of external helpers, particularly professional care givers, both allopathic and nonallopathic.

## Individual and Family Health Promotion Functions

The family is the human nest. Protection, nurturance, and education are its central functions, but its modalities are difficult to specify. Protection requires awareness and mediation; nurturance is achieved through love and caring; and education proceeds toward images and hopes for the future. These attributes are not easily converted to equivalencies in the language of professional care. Any attempt to do so invariably leaves out the interactive and continuous issue of family life-style. It is this webbing material of values, beliefs, expectations, criteria of choice, problem defining, problem solving, communication, and commitment that is unique to the family. The inadequacy of professional descriptions of these family functions is particularly obvious with regard to health care functions, as noted earlier. And within the health care domain of activity, those undertakings assignable as health-promoting functions are most difficult to account for beyond the simple health-promoting rituals of nutrition, hygiene, and the avoidance of environmental risks. Health promotion is both the process and the product of life-style. To isolate the health promotion strand in the life-style fabric is probably not possible or necessarily useful given the synergistic action of life-style. Research on life-style has been largely descriptive of a state or condition wherein certain behaviors variously influence the health of individuals. The works of Lester Breslow and N.B. Belloc, for example, supports the idea "that a lifetime of good health practices produces good health and extends the period of relatively good physical health status by some 30 years."[29] In effect, such studies affirm the overwhelming contribution of routine living to health promotion. It is odd, indeed, that the concept of health promotion as a primarily lay function needs such affirmation. Indeed, survey findings that report that less than 3 percent of the population seek good health from their doctors come as a surprise to health planners.[30] As Williams noted, "Everyone knows that health begins in the home. The problem is to get the health authorities, national and international, to realize it."[31]

There is a paucity of family research that pinpoints specific, purposeful health-promoting activities, in either professional or lay definitions of what these constitute. In Theodor Litman's overview of the literature on the family as a "basic unit in health and medical care," the scarcity of data on health care functions is apparent.[32] Falling back on his own studies of three-generational families, Litman establishes that health promotion and preventive practices dominate in contrast to the use of professional resources for these purposes (less than 1 percent) and that there are distinct generational differences in attitudes and beliefs regarding how to keep well. Little detail is available, however, on either the extent or the frequency of health-promoting procedures. Furthermore, there is little basis for assurance that activities defined as health promotion are in fact valid contributors to good health. Indeed, we are not even clear on the basis for reported positive effects of certain health-promoting practices. Certainly the placebo effect—belief that an activity *does* promote health—must be considered. It is clear that individuals and families operate within a belief structure about what causes disease and what they can do about it. Their concepts, however they might follow some mainstream beliefs about health promotion (on the order of the Breslow–Belloc health habits), can be substantially affected by social class, ethnic group, and regional variation.[33] Here the family's key role in health is simply to protect and nurture. Alert to its social setting, the family receives, interprets, and distributes information that it perceives as relevant to its security. Information with low salience is ignored, while threat-laden information mobilizes the family for appropriate protective action.[34] As a mediating agency on behalf of its members, the family communicates its presence and preferences to society, particularly to those structures that provide services essential for survival, acceptance, and happiness. Effective mediation to achieve those ends demands negotiation and compromise, sharing, and adaptation. There is clearly both cohesion and conflict involved, families in the community network sharing a common pool of health beliefs and practices and at the same time distinguishing their unique priorities, taboos, and life-styles. The cohesive areas of agreement on health behavior are perhaps taken for granted as the social norm, evidence of family variation (deviance) being more visible but of less overall consequence. Thus a Seventh Day Adventist family's conflict with the professional health care system on the matter of blood transfusion may obscure the larger areas of concordance. But the reality is that our knowledge of this process is primitive. There is no theoretical construction sufficiently generous to encompass the many forms of health communications, behaviors, and transactions; no observational strategy sufficiently sensitive and specific to achieve acceptable validity and reliability; and no analytic perspective sufficiently free of disciplinary bias to ensure balanced conclusions. We are, in effect, in the situation of having to infer the existence and power of the family's health mediating role from fragmentary evidence of intergenerational studies that provide some sense of the transmission of health traditions and their successive revisions.

Insufficiencies in our knowledge of the family's health role are most obvious with regard to health promotion and disease prevention. Some peripheral clues are available from anthropological studies describing cultural variations in beliefs about disease causation and effective prevention.[35] We know that primitive and folk beliefs exist in all cultures and that they can and do survive along with the acceptance of alternative scientific explanations.[36] We are less clear about their interaction and change. This issue is of special interest to our understanding of the family's function in health mediation. What is the extent and process of shifts in family health beliefs as these confront discordant community or scientific values? What factors of family structure or style influence these transactions? Research on behavior modification is helpful only in establishing the existence of resistance mechanisms and the formidable power of the family and individual structure of health beliefs. Studies of resistance to or compliance with professional advice are, however, of no help in illuminating the natural ongoing health belief transactions between the family and its external references. Health-promoting and disease-preventing activities as integral features of the *meaning* of family become health care artifacts of the nurturance and homemaking processes.[37] These processes have received considerable attention from anthropologists and health researchers. An important outcome of this interest has been the rationalization of living (social) functions as health activities subject to professional analysis and advice. In Irving Zola's term, certain family functions are medicalized—raised to consciousness as health/medical functions, which therefore become the legitimate concern (jurisdiction) of both families *and* health professionals.[38] This, in turn, has led to the construction of professional strategies for family health and the assignment of a professional nomenclature; birthing, bonding, parenting, and life style are examples. The implications of medicalization for the family as a mediating structure in health were discussed earlier. The point we wish to make now is that the health-promoting and disease-preventing functions of the family should be recognized as primary and dominant and have historically been beyond the effective control of professional interests.

If we can accept evidence of the family's profound role in health promotion and disease prevention, we must at the same time acknowledge variations in outcomes as measured by both family and professional criteria. There are several questions about this variation that must be addressed. The most fundamental issue here is, once again, what outcome criteria are appropriate in judging an individual or family's health-promoting and disease-preventing behavior? To date, the answer has been morbidity criteria, the frequency of episodes of symptoms, disease, social maladaptations, and injuries. Observations of these outcome criteria are professionally defined, although definitions may vary somewhat from study to study. Criteria that reflect levels of wellness, well-being, or positive health are absent, as are criteria that may be applied by individuals and families as measures of their own expectations and values. Such bias in judging lay effectiveness in health severely limits our perspective on those aspects of being and functioning that represent the continuous, instinctive process of what René Dubos has named "creative adaptation," the most profound process of health promotion and disease prevention.[39] By definition, the adaptive process will reflect individual (or family) perceptions of the situation, their interpretation of threat, their preferences for response, and their judgment of the efficacy of the response. Measurement of lay judgments of outcome against professional criteria may reveal disparities but not necessarily deficiencies in the adaptive process. This concept undoubtedly will present some difficulties for present strategies of health care evaluation. Professional tolerance for lay preferences in health methods or outcomes can be expected to remain low. Deviant behavior in health-promoting and disease-preventing practices will remain the target of professional health education efforts designed to launder indigenous practices and replace them with professional techniques. This may pertain even under circumstances where evidence indicates that the deviant practice is reasonable and beneficial for a particular social group.[40]

## Healing, Curing, Caring

When it comes to the matter of intervening in the disease process, managing injuries, or caring in the illness state, the perspective on the lay role is less benign. Even though the physiological response to the insult of disease or injury is acknowledged and the responsibility of the individual to cooperate in the healing and restorative process often reaches the level of exhortation,[41] the demarcation between internal and external control has been politicized as a jurisdictional issue, that is, lay versus professional. The debate on family functions in healing, curing, and caring has two dominant themes. There is, first, the central concern with the efficacy of such practices. So-called primitive and folk health practices have been elaborately described by anthropologists, defended through testimonials, rationalized, and codified, or criticized as dangerous, ineffective, placebo, or nuisance (delaying seeking professional care or interfering with professional advice). The matter of efficacy is further compounded by the degree of fit of an indigenous health care practice with dominant allopathic values. Each system of practice has its own criteria for judging effectiveness; yet the validation criteria of allopathic medicine have been universally applied.

A second aspect of the family or lay health care debate is certainly tied to the issue of efficacy, in the sense that the concern for safety is a factor in deciding *who* should administer the care. Safety is a concept that reveals itself as a complex of other issues, including the notion of relativity (safer than what?); qualifications of the provider (experience, sensitivity); potential for side effects (iatrogenesis, false negatives); and audit and accountability (the presence or absence of external review).

For reasons noted earlier, we must approach existing research on self-care with caution. Variations in study populations, definitions, and methods make generalizations hazardous. Or perhaps one could look at it the other way and say that general impressions are more useful than specific findings standing alone. It is at least helpful at this stage of our knowledge to have an overall grasp of the magnitude of self-care activity, particularly those undertakings intended to deal with sickness and injury. This is the area of self-care that is the focus of both lay and professional attention and in which the shift in locus of control from professional to lay person is most obvious, most active, and most controversial.

A more than academic interest in lay self-care emerged in the United Kingdom as a result, ironically, of the establishment of the National Health Service (NHS). The NHS made available and accessible a universal primary professional resource, the practitioner of general medicine. This front line of primary medical care became an effective response to public demand for primary care services and at the same time an incentive to both practitioner and patient *to use* those services. In other words, the general practice structure is in the position of both meeting and stimulating demands for medical care. The result, predictably, was heavy but variable use of the general practitioner as direct provider and as gatekeeper to secondary (consultant, hospital) care resources. This raised questions about the efficient use of the NHS and, specifically, the possibility that it was creating an unproductive and possibly counterproductive public response. The theory was postulated that increasing lay self-care competence could result in more efficacious use of professional providers of care. Thus the stage was set for piecing together extant research on the level and distribution of self-care practices in the United Kingdom as a basis for planning its further nurturance. An independent working party chaired by a prominent general practitioner, John Fry, determined on the basis of available evidence that active self-care constitutes 63 percent of *all* disease/illness care interventions and that an additional 16 percent of such episodes are also self-controlled, but through the device of not taking any action.[42] Dr. Fry and his colleagues concluded from their review: "Self care is an inevitable, important, but almost totally neglected level of care in all systems of health care. . . . Without self care any system of health care would be swamped."[43] The working party report offered several recommendations for research on self-care to determine its specific "nature, content and outcome . . . and to define and encourage all that is good in self-care."[44]

Several aspects of self-care of special interest emerge from the British report. The most surprising, perhaps, is the high level of self-care practice in the context of a nationalized health service system. Clearly, this argues against the conventional wisdom that self-care can be expected to operate at high levels only as compensation for a lack of professional care resources. The only cross-national study that compares self-care levels appears to corroborate the view that the organization of professional services seems not to be related to self-care activity.[45] Less is known, of course, about the levels of self-care in the developing countries, where access to professional services is more difficult to define and account for, given that the bulk of professional care is provided by indigenous healers who are not registered or regulated. The level of self-care activity relative to professional care could be construed as an important indication of one attribute of its efficacy, namely social and cultural acceptability.

Reviews of studies made in the United States establish the self-care baseline for minor illness and injury at a uniformly high level.[46] The research of Klaus Roghmann and Robert Haggerty is an example.[47] Their findings were based on information collected from daily diaries maintained by a random sample of 512 families in upstate New York. A 28-day period yielded data on 71,316 person-days of health experience and associated activities. More than 90 percent of the health actions taken were based on self-decision. Of more than 11,000 person-days in which there was a complaint, only sixteen families reported that advice had been received from health professionals. The proportion of no action self-care fell between 15 and 17 percent, a figure nearly identical with the British findings.[48]

There is little doubt that self-care activity in countries where data are available is by far the dominant mode of care for minor illness and injury. But another interesting point revealed by both British and American studies is the prominence of medicine taking in the mix of self-care. A 1972 Food and Drug Administration (FDA) survey of health practices and opinions of Americans gave special emphasis to the medicine-taking aspect of self-care. This study highlighted the public practice of "taking something" in the belief that it promotes health, prevents disease, eases symptoms, or cures a health problem. These medication practices include use of vitamins and nutritional supplements, health foods, weight control medications, medications for both common and serious ailments, aids to stop smoking, and medications for arthritis/rheumatism and cancer.[49] Pratt summarized additional research that established the importance of medication as "one of the major forms of health care activity" and self-medication (nonprescription) as a preeminent form of self-care activity.[50] The sheer amount of medicine being ingested is certainly sufficient grounds for raising the question of the efficacy of this aspect of self-care. There is, for example, the potential for crossover among medications and all the problems inherent in the medicine hoarding process,[51] such as wastage, spoilage, and loss of potency, use by various family members, and memory failure regarding the purpose of a particular medication.

The amount of nonprescription medications may be related to socioeconomic status, the more affluent and better educated purchasing more of them.[52] This appears to run contrary to conventional wisdom that nonprescription self-medication is an attractive option for those who cannot afford, or do not have access to, or do not appreciate the efficacy of, prescribed drugs. It may well be that families of lower socioeconomic status have less access to over-the-counter drugs as well as prescribed drugs; indeed they have been found to have fewer of both.[53] At the same time, the widespread popularity of over-the-counter items suggests that level of sophistication with regard to health knowledge is not a factor. Indeed, a study by David and Deanne Knapp of self-medication in the United States revealed that knowledge of medications was "respectable" among users.[54] The purchase of over-the-counter items is apparently not a mindless activity and, further, a preferred choice among choices. In looking at this question of the relation of education to self-care practices, including self-medication, on a global basis, Stella Quah notes that her research in Singapore agrees with the findings of others elsewhere that "these tendencies appear stronger among educated people."[55]

Self-medication is certainly the most researched aspect of self-care for minor illness and injury, but the wide range of other such activities deserves mention and further study: first aid for minor injuries, cuts, scrapes, bruises, and burns; vaporizers and bed rest for colds and flu; ointments, compresses, and astringents for skin problems; home surgery for blisters and splinters; kisses and Band-aids for imaginary "boo-boos"; massage and hot tub baths for sore muscles; chicken noodle soup and a "nice hot cup of tea" for anything; hot water bottles and heating pads for menstrual cramps; ice packs for swellings; vinegar douches and yogurt for vaginal infections; hydrogen peroxide for ear wax; salt water gargles—the list could go on and on. In addition to these treatments, certain items of diagnostic and monitoring equipment are increasingly found in home use, such as thermometers, sphygmomanometers, otoscopes, home throat culture and urine-testing kits, and home pregnancy tests. Given the current trend, one can expect increased testing and marketing of a wide range of other intermediate health care technologies.

In effect, the test of efficacy of self-care for minor illness and symptom relief, if judged by the pervasiveness and sweep of its practice across social, ethnic, and cultural groups, must give special weight to the notion of *acceptability* as positive evidence. It is a reflection of belief in the utility of self-care based on the commonly experienced self-limiting nature of most minor illnesses. There is also the obvious efficiency factor in self-care; being able to take immediate action without going through the time- and cost-laden rituals of the professional health care bureaucracy. Efficiency is also enhanced through the elimination of any requirement to interpret the decisions or actions of others on an individual's behalf. It is a self-contained system of symptom recognition, interpretation and assessment, treatment, and evaluation of effectiveness.

External measures of efficacy of self-care in healing, curing, and caring activities, apart from the arguments of common practice, custom, and the socially acknowledged preference (and benefits) of self-control in personal health care, are less available than studies of the extent of self-care practices. Two studies that attempted to focus on both the amount and the efficacy of such practices are unfortunately limited in their generalizability. Both were undertaken by general practitioners who surveyed their patients. The work of C.P. Elliot-Binns[56] in Britain and Paol Pederson[57] in Denmark asked the dual questions of how much self-care preceded a visit to the doctor and how relevant the self-care was. Findings of the two studies were remarkably comparable, each suggesting that the vast proportion of self-care undertakings were relevant or at the very least neither helpful nor harmful.[a] But neither these two studies nor others available at this time address the matter of the efficacy of self-care in terms of its mediating benefits. John Williamson and Kate Danaher, however, in their review of the state of self-care activity, posit that the decision-making aspect of self-care, lay referral (seeking advice from relatives, friends), is important "in

a. In fact, it may even be discovered that the very notion of the self-limitation of most minor illness and injury depends on a certain level of lay self-care competence that has always been in place and prevented further complications. For example, children's scrapes may easily develop into far more serious infections if not given proper attention. Thus the category of self-limiting illness is broadened by unacknowledged self-care practices.

its abilities both to suggest the most relevant source of treatment and to recommend the objectives to be met."[58]

Similarly, it is reasonable to look at other aspects of self-care as preferred options to professional care, particularly when that care is viewed as unsatisfactory. Pearl German, in her study of the health behavior of an aged population, noted a trend in her data that suggests a "tendency . . . for greater percentages of individuals to purchase over-the-counter drugs when they rated their medical care as poor/fair."[59] Thus an important mediating aspect of self-care is its value as an option to professional care. In this sense mediation is an adaptive process, responding to exigencies of the external health resource, its quality, and its availability.[60]

The more profound mediating functions of self-care are expressed in the diffusion of lay self-care competence in the ordinary activities of perceiving health norms, self-monitoring against criteria of normal health, interpreting symptoms, and deciding what, if any, health action to take. This involves a highly complex and only marginally understood process of integrating and interpreting evidence and weighing the cost-benefit-liability ratios of various professional and self-care alternatives in cure or care. Mediating activities are an amalgam of culture and class, learned through socialization and continuously tested and adjusted through experience with disease itself.[61]

In contrast, the contribution of formally learned cure and care skills can be presumed negligible given the low status, poor quality, and low availability of health education for children as well as adults. Furthermore, organized health education programs have emphasized primary prevention, to a modest degree symptom recognition, and only rarely and in narrow terms curing disease and caring for illness (that is, patient education). Organized self-care education is too recent and too limited a development to expect an important impact on society at this time. What the public has learned *systematically* about approaches to medical intervention it has learned from the widely available lay-oriented medical literature.[62] Aside from the more diffuse mediating benefits of self-care competence and confidence in that competence (empowerment), there are areas of technology that more directly protect and nurture the individual's integrity in personal health care. Several have been known as important professional strategies in health care, but only recently have they been recognized as valuable in self-care. One of these is the personal health history.

The personal medical history and record is probably the most useful tool in health and medical care. It can provide the basis for identifying factors influencing and defining health status, clarifying and ordering problems, planning interventions, and monitoring programs. Designed as problem oriented, the medical record can not only enhance the efficacy of medical care but also control iatrogenic effects related to errors in the medical assessment–decision-making process. Such a Problem Oriented Medical Record (POMR) was developed by Lawrence Weed, but its adoption by hospitals and physicians has been slow.[63] Weed has also published a version of POMR for the lay person. In the introduction to the POMR manual of instruction, a "Layperson's Statement" gives particular emphasis to the mediating benefits to individuals in maintaining their own POMR. Ruth Page has stressed:

> The patient's medical record becomes the patient's passport into the medical system; it carries him from one facet to another without repetition or time-wasting, it keeps him informed about every detail of his own health care. For he is the one who must carry it in his hands; he is the source, the only link in the chain that can be coupled to every other link. . . . He doesn't feel stupid because all is explained to him as keeper of the record, and he is a full participant in all his health care.[64]

The efficacy of self-care as a mediating resource is related to an individual's ability to control information about health status, disease risk, and the medical care process. The POMR and other devices designed to help individuals and families organize information about their health have been available in many forms, including the special place in the family Bible for births and deaths. The extent of lay health record keeping is unknown. Some research has shown who makes family health decisions, how they are arrived at, and under what circumstances, but there has been only scant attention to the process of organizing and storing health information as a data base for planning health actions and engaging the professional care system in a self-protecting way.[b] At this time we can

---

b. Family record keeping has been of interest to researchers seeking continuous data on family health behavior. Health diaries and other lay-managed recording procedures have been used for this purpose, but they are not intended as systematic family-controlled records for purposes of lay participation in health care management.

only speculate on the contribution of information control in the mix of self-care benefits to health mediation.

In summary, we can offer the generalization that self-care by individuals and families is a substantial proportion of all health care activity, is characteristic of many cultures, and appears to meet standards of efficacy as defined by expected benefits (symptom relief in situations of self-limiting illness), safety (as relative to "no action" or professional care), and efficiency (ease of access to self, over-the-counter drugs, and so forth) and costs (related to professional care or restricted medications). There is a good deal of room for careful evaluation of these attributes of lay self-care, but its constitution as the base of the health care pyramid is undeniable. And for good or for bad, it joins environmental and economic factors as a major determinant of both health status and the need for and use of the professional component of the health care system.

Nowhere is the lay contribution to health care so obvious as in the management of chronic disease. Here the historical precedent is established and its benefits confirmed, both for adults and for children.[65] Self-administered diabetes care is, of course, the classic example. But many other chronic conditions have been found to be not only amenable to self or family care but significantly benefited by the involvement of the patient and the family. Stroke is a case in point. In a retrospective study of patients who had a diagnosed cardiovascular accident with partial paralysis, it was found that the benefits of the initial rehabilitation phase were maintained and sometimes improved two to twelve years later. Moreover, the researchers concluded, "The rehabilitative status of the patient was maintained as well through education of the rehabilitant and his family as through the use of public health nursing and community resources in the majority of cases."[66] Other chronic conditions, once assumed to depend almost totally on professional (indeed institutional) care, are being reassessed as more efficaciously cared for by the patient and family. David Agle, in commenting on this trend with regard to hemophilia, noted that many advocates of home management, "both physician and laymen, are highly enthusiastic. Some consider it a major breakthrough, akin to the provision of insulin for the diabetic."[67] Arguments in support of this view include its contribution to the promotion of patient autonomy and independence, a "normalization of life activities . . . decrease in school

and work absenteeism . . . shorter time in formal medical treatment . . . decreases time in sick role . . . positive influence on the
emotional state of the patient and his family . . . decrease in . . .
fear, anger, anxiety, depression, and helplessness . . . increase in
positive self-regard . . . and a sense of personal gain achieved through
the home care program." These claimed benefits as well as possible
areas of counterproductivity (such as relinquishment of physician
responsibility, potential for errors in family judgment, and promoting a "smothering" of the patient by the family care givers) have
not been sufficiently studied. It is clear that there is a need for
research on the question of how to arrive at the most efficacious
mix of professional service and self-care. To answer this question
will require accounting for the full range of benefits, both bio-
medical and social, and the contribution of patients and their families in setting criteria.

The family's explanation of disease causation will certainly vary
by both culture[68] and social class, although as Ruth Elder cautions,
some of the differences (at least as related to social class) may
moderate as a function of generally rising educational levels and
other assimilating social changes.[69] Similarly, notions of susceptibility, perceived seriousness, personal concern about a given disease,
sense of personal control in prevention, and view of what can be
done to cure the disease are related to life circumstances.[70] There
is less clarity, however, with regard to variations in family treatment
or management of all classes of disease, particularly chronic disease.
Indeed, some disease, viewed as the necessary consequence of aging
or a particular life-style or the inevitable result of poverty or certain
hazardous occupations may not be labeled disease, at least not in
the ordinary sense of causing the family to alter the normal relationships of its members. How, and *if*, treatment for the chronically
ill is perceived by families and the nature of its character and rationalization are still vague.

The dominant theories of family health behavior reflect the
essentially Parsonian view of the family as increasingly incompetent
to cope effectively with illness of long duration without serious
consequences of discordance, disaffection, general deterioration
of its integrity, and ultimate negative impact on the welfare of the
chronically ill family member. Within this construction of reality,
one can explain the progress of incompetence from its reaction to

the "acute stage," the "reconstruction stage," the "plateau stage," and, finally, the "deteriorative stage."[71] Each stage of disease, the theory asserts, takes its toll of the family's emotional reserve. There are, of course, suggestions for strengthening the family role at each stage through family education and professional medical support.

With nearly 50 percent of the civilian population of the United States having one or more chronic diseases and a substantial proportion of the bedfast elderly living at home, we can at the very least assume that support of the chronically ill is a normative function of families.[72] In this sense the presence of health deviance serves to stimulate the awareness of family membership and focus family action. The question of the effect of chronic illness on family solidarity is a complex one with evidence running in both directions. Litman's review of research on the impact of chronic illness on family relations concluded that

> most illnesses reportedly had little effect on family solidarity, an equal number appeared to have either brought the family together or made their relationship more difficult . . .
>
>   . . . there were fairly marked generational differences [where] a member's illness in the parent generation tended to have a more integrating effect on the family [while] the opposite was true for their married children.
>
>   . . . on the whole, acute conditions were less likely to have affected family relations than the more serious chronic ones.
>
>   . . . on the other hand, there appeared to be a direct relationship between severity of the family's illness and its impact on the family's relations.
>
>   . . . Families whose members were considered to be seriously ill . . . were about equally likely to have been brought closer together as driven further apart.[73]

The fact remains that families are heavily and increasingly involved with chronic disease management with self-evident success, as measured in the relatively low proportion of hospitalization versus home care for even major disabling conditions. Less than 5 percent of adults with chronic diseases are institutionalized.[74] In contrast with the impact of an acute illness or injury, the onset of some chronic diseases is gradual, offering families an opportunity to adapt almost imperceptively to consequential disabilities. Similarly, a prolonged period of convalescence after an initial crisis may moderate the impact of the illness on the family's coping resources even to the point of nurturing family stability.[75] While assistance in managing chronic illness continues to flow from extended families, friendship networks, and other mediating resources external to the family, the family itself remains the dominant care giver.[76] Coping styles vary by culture, class, personal attributes of the ill person, and perhaps the nature of the family's conjugal organization, although the latter has not been specifically studied with regard to chronic disease.[77] The family's previous experience of illness is likely to be an especially important influence on coping style as well as effectiveness, but once again research is meager on this point. Further, little is known about variations in coping styles as influenced by a family's access to technical knowledge or how it is more generally connected to the community pattern of adopting new practices.

The characteristic of the family most germane to its function in chronic disease is its ability to provide continuity of care, a commitment that allows the person with the illness to count on this support in interpreting the implications of the illness and in providing the reassurance necessary to focus and sustain the patient's motivation for adaptation or recovery. There is considerable room for speculation on how and why family service to the chronically ill is effective and in what ways it may fail. Research to date offers an overview of the complex factors involved and interacting. There still remain, however, unanswered questions about the family's role in information gathering, communication, interpretation, and decision making as these help the patient orient herself to the reality of her status and her potential for rehabilitation.

By and large, research on the family and chronic disease has been fragmentary, theory-free, and anarchic when it comes to definitions and populations studied. Furthermore, most studies focus on either demographic factors (family size, severity of illness, family illness history, social class) or psychosocial aspects of family life (family solidarity, health knowledge and beliefs, caring strategies). An integrated, systematic approach is needed. But there is an equally pressing requirement that research undertaken in this area be sensitive to lay definitions of the care process.

We have thus described the family's health care function in both its instrumental and its expressive aspects. It is important now to look at a special instance of family health care function that illumines historical and current conditions of health practice and raises, more specifically, issues relevant to the interface of professional and lay health care. We have chosen to look at childbirth, not because it is typical of current family health care but because it constitutes such a rich case history. The historical changes in the practice of childbirth in America contain nearly all the elements of the critique of American medicine presented in Chapter 1. In the course of this century, childbirth has changed from a life event that invariably took place at home to a medically managed condition that occurs almost exclusively in hospitals. We have tried to provide some of the details of this rather dramatic example of medicalization to show that the process is not simple but results from the multiple interests of families and the medical profession. A second major element of the critique we presented was that medical treatment often produces its own ill effects, both physical and social. This has certainly been true in childbirth, as both the popular and the scientific literature recognize. We have reviewed this critique for two reasons. First, the critique of the hazards of medical childbirth is a critique by mediating structures themselves, both single families and the loosely organized home birth movement. This critique is not an academic one, because it actually informs personal decisions. The second reason for our attention to the subject is that it illustrates what happens when a health care activity is removed from the family's jurisdiction. The critique is not only *by* mediating structures, it is about mediating structures and the damage that can be done to the social bonds that make them up. Families are created in childbirth. The home birth movement is quite self-consciously trying to make childbirth safe for families.

## A CLOSER LOOK: HOME CHILDBIRTH

Childbirth at home is probably the most dramatic example of a mediating structure's self-care activity. A growing questioning of the assumption that hospitals are the most appropriate and desirable place for normal childbearing may also be the self-care strategy that is most threatening to hospitals and the medical profession, judging from their denunciations of it. Any appreciable increase in the proportion of births occurring in the home does constitute a significant economic threat to hospitals, especially as the birthrate continues to drop. It will be interesting to see how hospitals respond to this gathering consumer movement and whether or not their maternity wards become more homelike.

There is a burgeoning popular and scientific literature criticizing the common practices of hospital childbirth. Many of these criticisms have as their agenda the promotion of one or another alternative birthplace, the most common of which is the home. The home birth literature is usually written for a popular audience, for people who are and will be having babies. Although the enthusiasm for the home birth experience is common to all members of the movement, their interests differ considerably, as do their perspectives on the problems of hospital obstetrics. Feminists see childbirth practices preempted from women by a male-dominated medical profession; counterculture members see the human body as the prisoner of technology; midwives see the professional issues inherent in the takeover of normal childbirth by medical obstetrics. A mediating structures perspective, which we will employ, examines the historical and recent changes in the practice of childbirth from the family's point of view.

## From Social Childbirth to the Obstetrical Ward

Babies have not always been born in hospitals. In colonial America the birth of a child was a major social event in the home, an occasion for extended and usually happy visiting with relatives. Birth was the exclusive province of women; within the family, mothers, sisters, cousins, and aunts would be present at the birth to lend the support of experience or learn what it would be like when their turn came. Such gatherings, which lasted through labor, birth, and postpartum care, were common throughout the eighteenth and nineteenth centuries, even when male doctors, rather than midwives, began delivering the babies. Before the twentieth century, the majority of American births took place at home, in the mother's bed. Women's experience of childbirth was thus profoundly family centered. Not only did they give birth in their own homes, but it was during just these times that they saw the most of their female relatives. The midwife's role in the birth was primarily passive; she remained with the mother throughout labor and delivery, providing words of comfort, traditional folk medicines, warm compresses, and glasses of wine. Midwives rarely used forceps or anesthesia, the new instruments of the obstetrical trade.[78]

A precondition for the hospitalization of childbirth was the growth of the medical specialty of obstetrics, an interesting chapter in the history of the medical profession. Obstetrics was one of the last areas of medicine to gain professional recognition; as late as 1910, 50 percent of births in the United States were attended by midwives.[79] The problem for obstetrics was that the majority of both doctors and midwives regarded childbirth as a normal event, not a sickness. Add to this the fact that obstetricians were men and that childbirth had always been regarded as the province of women, and it becomes clear that the event had to undergo some significant redefinition before the change in birth attendants could take place. Obstetricians began to argue that "normal" pregnancy and birth were uncommon and that every woman should have medical supervision to be prepared for any complications that might develop. In the new medical thinking about childbirth, nature became less and less adequate, more apt to be improved by intervention. During this period of transition, women had some choice over the kind of birth attendant they wanted. But since doctors were considerably more expensive than midwives, there were clear class factors at work in the choice; midwifery in 1910 was concentrated among immigrant groups in the urban Northeast and among poor blacks in the South.[80]

Once birth began to be regarded as a medical event, the home became a less appropriate place for it. Whereas in 1900 less than 5 percent of women delivered in hospitals, by 1939 over half did so.[81] The percentage of hospital births reached an apparent peak in 1973, at 99.3 percent, and has declined somewhat since then (99.0 percent in 1978).[82]

What were the causes of this rapid acceptance of hospital childbirth? Perhaps the most straightforward reason was the introduction of anesthesia, which was available only in hospitals. A technique called twilight sleep, which consisted of injections of morphine and an amnesiac drug called scopalomine, was developed in Germany around the turn of the century. Though the morphine did dull the pain somewhat, the drug's effectiveness lay in the fact that the woman remembered nothing of her experience. The technique was not immediately well received by the predominantly male medical profession, many of whom continued to believe that it was a woman's lot to suffer in childbirth, but the idea of a painless childbirth quickly became popular with the childbearing public. The method was first widely used by wealthy women, and some, like Mrs. John Jacob Astor, even organized campaigns to promote its use. By the 1930s twilight sleep had become accepted medical practice in hospitals. Doctors soon found that the drugs made women more manageable during labor and delivery and more amenable to other interventions.[83]

The overall issue, then, was one of control. The hospital was a place where the difficult, sometimes dangerous business of giving birth could be managed efficiently and safely. It was simply the modern thing to do; as Rose Kennedy remarked, "the fashion changed."[84] And as a result, women began to get some psychological distance from their own bodies. Because they were able to give birth without any consciousness whatever of the pain women had always and frequently had to bear, they must have felt an exhilarating sense of freedom and a heady sense of control over their own bodies.

But it was not only control over their pain that women sought in the hospital. By the 1930s the maternity hospital was also perceived as the safest possible place to give birth, far from the "household germs" written about in the women's magazines of the 1920s.[85] The popular culture germ theory of disease made women insecure about how clean their homes were, no matter how many of the new cleaning products they bought and used. Hospitals, on the other hand, were pictured as bastions of white-enameled sanitation. Furthermore, the hospital's equipment included all the X-ray machines, laboratories, blood banks, and incubators for premature infants, in case of complications. In fact, it was not their own safety women sought in the hospital so much as it was the safety of their infants. Neonatal mortality rates have always greatly exceeded maternal mortality rates; in 1939, the year of the 50 percent hospitalization for birth, the national maternal mortality rate was 40.4/10,000, and the neonatal mortality rate was 29.3/1,000.[86] Support for the perception that hospital births really were safer for mothers and infants came from the continuously declining mortality rates and increasing hospitalization of birth. The fallacy of this correlation will be pointed out later, but these trends are still cited as reasons for attempting to achieve 100 percent hospitalization for birth.[87]

Another concern of the 1930s that tended to increase hospitalization of birth was the declining birthrate. This affected mothers and doctors in different ways, but both saw hospitalization as an answer. For mothers the declining birthrate meant fewer children, which naturally increased concern for the safety of the infants that were born. Because mothers had fewer birth experiences, each one became more significant and special, and they could better afford the increased costs of the hospital. Further, the introduction of maternity clothes and bottle feeding at the turn of the century also contributed considerably to women's freedom from confinement in the home. On the other hand, obstetricians, who were alarmed at the decline in the birthrate, especially among their clients, the upper classes, saw painless, hospitalized childbirth as a way to encourage these women to have more children.[88] The hospital, then, was conceived of as the modern, safe place to give birth, admirably suited to the different but coinciding needs of the modern woman and her doctor.[89]

If mothers felt that they were gaining some control over their birth pain and their safety by going to the hospital to give birth, it was at the price of giving doctors control over them. Women who labored and delivered in hospitals, away from friends and family, were surrounded by professional strangers and largely or completely in their control, depending on the amount of anesthesia they received. In contrast to the midwife, who had no instruments or drugs with which to intervene and who thus had to rely on time, social support, and herbal remedies, the doctor by the 1930s had the most powerful tools of modern obstetrics: anesthesia, analgesia, and forceps.

Many writers have noted the "technological imperative" of modern medicine, which impels doctors to do all they have been trained to do, and hospitalized childbirth is a superb example of this.[90] As one doctor put it, "It is very difficult for a person trained in technical know-how to do technically nothing during a normal birth."[91] The history of obstetrics has been and continues to be the history of interference in the birth process, sometimes, but not always, with good effects.

Even at the clinical level, the hospitalization of birth has not been an uncomplicated story of medical progress. Since the days of the epidemics of childbed fever common to European and American lying-in hospitals, the hospitalization of childbirth has been accompanied by iatrogenic effects, both clinical and social. A famous study by the New York Academy of Medicine of maternal mortality in New York City compared the relative safety of home and hospital birth.[92] It found that for the years 1930–32, there were 1.9/1,000 maternal deaths at home, compared with 4.5/1,000 in hospitals. More women died in hospitals both from infection and from hemorrhage. A national study of the same period, the report of the White House Conference on Child Health and Family Protection, found that overall maternal mortality rates had not declined from 1915 to 1930, despite increased medical care. Furthermore, the report found that infant death from birth injuries, reflecting the increasing use of forceps in hospital delivery, had actually increased by 40 to 50 percent in the same period.[93]

Since 1935, however, maternal and infant mortality rates have steadily declined, even as hospitalization of birth has approached 100 percent, leading many advocates to draw a causal connection between the two. But as A.L. Cochrane writes, "this sort of correlation is not evidence."[94] To illustrate his point, he juxtaposes two charts, one showing declining maternal and infant mortality rates and increasing hospitalization, the other showing declining maternal and infant mortality rates and declining length of stay in hospitals after birth.[95] Devitt's study concludes that hospital obstetric care did not benefit healthy women with normal pregnancies in the period 1930–60.[96]

The real issue today, however, is no longer the maternal mortality rate, which is now happily reduced, but the infant mortality rate, which has not declined nearly as much. American infant mortality statistics are, in George Silver's phrase, "worse than a scandal."[97] The 1976 infant death rate of 15.1/1,000 ranked eighteenth among developed countries, trailing Sweden, the Netherlands, Japan, New Zealand, Singapore, Ireland, Hong Kong, and many others.[98] Furthermore, the infant mortality rates of these countries, except for Sweden, have been decreasing faster than the U.S. rate. The evidence is overwhelming that the key to improving infant mortality statistics is to improve prenatal care, especially to poor women who have a disproportionate share of low-birth-weight infants.[99] Yet the emphasis in American medical research and practice has been and continues to be on correcting problems at birth and after, as illustrated by the mushrooming of neonatology units, rather than preventing the problems in the first place.

As we have seen, during the twentieth century, birth has come to be defined as a medical event, meaning that it rarely takes place without some sort of medical management. According to Rebecca Parfitt, only 10 percent of all labors in the United States proceed without some level of obstetric intervention.[100] The other 90 percent of mothers experience what has been referred to as "just in case obstetrics,"[101] "operative furor,"[102] and a "cascade of interventions."[103] The term "cascade" is particularly apt because it conveys the sense of a stream of connected medical acts, one of which leads directly to the next.

Medical interventions in childbirth frequently begin before labor itself begins. Contractions may be induced through chemical or mechanical means so that delivery will occur at a time that is convenient for doctor or mother, a technique that has been growing in popularity.[104] The same hormones used to start labor may also be used to speed it up if it is not progressing well enough on its own. This is very common practice; in one large urban teaching hospital during the year 1973, almost half of all mothers had their labor stimulated.[105] In the hospital Nancy Shaw studied, it was routine for all first mothers.[106] The precise effects of these hormones on the unborn baby are unknown but suspect. Their effect on the mother, however, has been frequently observed: they make her contractions faster and stronger, sometimes so suddenly as to cause her great distress.[107] Frequently women who had been managing their labor until this point with breathing and relaxation alone find themselves unable to handle the new, suddenly stronger contractions and request more drugs to help them deal with the pain. Recent figures on the percentage of women delivering in hospitals who receive some form of anesthesia vary; in all cases it is more than half. Lewis Mehl's sample of low-risk hospital births showed a combined total of 76.8 percent receiving anesthesia.[108] A national survey of hospital births done in 1970 by the American College of Obstetricians and Gynecologists gathered information from 80 percent of the hospitals in the United States; 82 percent of them reported that *almost all* (80–100 percent) of their patients received medication for pain during labor or delivery, and 81 percent said that almost all (80–100 percent) of their patients had anesthesia.[109] These drugs render women passive, effectively reducing their already limited control over the situation. And they make even more interventions necessary, such as the fetal heart monitor, so that the effects of medication on the fetus can be closely watched.

For women who have been given drugs or who are being monitored, the flat-on-the-back, even strapped-down position is routine. Such a position makes labor difficult because it forces the uterus to work against gravity. It may increase the woman's blood pressure and will certainly increase the need for an episiotomy, the cut doctors make in the floor of the pelvis so the birth outlet will be bigger.[110] Such incisions are rarely necessary when women deliver in any other position. In one Boston hospital for the year 1973, 77 percent of mothers had episiotomies, and 27 percent required forceps to assist delivery.[111] Nationally, rates of episiotomies have been estimated at 70 percent; in England the rate is 15 percent, and in Holland it is 8 percent.[112] Episiotomy is a much rarer phenomenon in midwife-assisted deliveries, as is the supine position.

The effects on the fetus of all these interventions are only beginning to be understood. For a long time it was thought that the placenta, which circulates the mother's blood to the fetus, acted as a kind of barrier to filter any toxins from the blood circulated to the fetus, but recent research has proved this belief completely false.[113] Any drugs that enter the mother's bloodstream circulate to the fetus. From there they may return to the mother (before the umbilical cord is cut), or they may be metabolized and eliminated by the newborn after birth. The elimination of these drugs by the neonate is very slow because the newborn's liver is not fully developed. The presence of these drugs, then, may aggravate jaundice, a common condition of newborns.[114] Furthermore, all pain-relieving drugs alter or depress the respiratory functions of neonates, a serious problem, since oxygen deprivation is the newborn's point of greatest vulnerability.[115] Other neonatal responses to drugs are bluish extremities, mucus-blocked breathing passages, reduced alertness and reactivity, delayed sucking response, and reduced smiling, all of which have further consequences that will be examined later.[116]

These clinical iatrogenic effects of medical interventions in the birth process are unfortunately not isolated or unusual. One medical intervention tends to lead directly to another, in what has been called a "medical carousel." Mehl's study of two matched populations of mothers having home and hospital deliveries showed significant differences in the number of complications of labor and delivery, neonatal complications, and procedures used. There was significantly more fetal distress, elevated blood pressure, bleeding, birth injuries, neonatal infection, and respiratory distress among the hospital mothers when all other factors were controlled for. There were also significantly more hormone injections, forceps deliveries, Caesarean sections, episiotomies, anesthesia, and analgesia in the hospital.[117] Of course, not all these techniques are performed on every woman who gives birth in a hospital. But as has been repeatedly confirmed, the correlations between interventions are very high.

So are the costs. No discussion of hospital birth would be complete without mention of its cost. In New York City the cost of private maternity care ranges upwards of $2,000 for a normal, uncomplicated delivery and a three-day hospital stay. Doctors' fees alone frequently run to $700 or more.[118] In California hospital costs in 1977 averaged $1,150 to $1,550.[119] Certainly many families have health insurance to help meet these costs; but policies frequently exclude from coverage prenatal complications, the first few days of the infant's life, and pregnancies begun before the policy takes effect or even up to eleven months after, and maternity care is often only partially covered. By almost anyone's standards, having a baby in a hospital is an expensive undertaking.

Hospitalized childbirth is another case in which modern medicine has had the tragic effect of attenuating people's abilities to deal with pain and illness in unique and autonomous ways. We have already seen some of the clinical manifestations of medically produced ill health through interference in an event not even thought of as an illness until the late nineteenth century. The medicalization of normal childbirth, in fact, may be the paradigmatic situation of medically created and complicated disease. But its ill effects are not only, or even mostly, physical. We will look later at evidence that suggests that the medical practice of childbirth does at least temporary and possibly permanent damage to the most fundamental of social bonds, those between infants and their parents.

Before the baby is born, however, the social relationship which comes under attack is that of the mother and father. Hospitals have traditionally banned the new father from both labor and delivery rooms. Although the precedent for the exclusion of the father from the lying-in room clearly goes back a long way, the modern exclusion of the father places the woman entirely in the hands of strange nurses and her usually male obstetrician, not the female members of her family.[120] This is unlike any other culture's approach to labor and birth.[121] Admittedly, the situation has been changing, as hospitals have realized that allowing fathers in labor rooms reduces demands on the nursing staff, but many hospitals still ban fathers from delivery rooms. One hospital in California called the police to forcibly remove a young man who had chained himself to his wife's labor bed.[122] The issue is clearly one of hospital convenience, not medical necessity. The birth of twins in a Boston hospital brought twenty-two people into the delivery room to watch, despite the mother's objection. "She asked, 'Can all these people come and watch and my husband can't?'"[123]

Possibly more than at any other time in her life, a woman will need assistance and comfort during childbirth. Yet this is exactly what is most effectively denied her. It is easy to see that the lack of privacy in the hospital could be distressing to some women. But more than just privacy, a laboring woman needs one person to be with her throughout the entire labor and delivery, someone who can help her integrate this highly intense and intimate experience into the rest of her life. Ideally, of course, this person should be the father of the child.

Hospital personnel change shifts every eight hours. Maternity ward residents, nurses, and aides see babies being born every day; they cannot possibly be expected to share fully the intensity of each woman's experience. Medical personnel cannot *care* for a woman as her family would. They do not love her, and it is not reasonable to expect that they should. It would be quite unfair to attack the hospital staff for failing to provide enough emotional support to women in labor; though some may indeed have the inclination, none has the time to sit quietly with a woman through the long hours of labor.

The attention they do have to give her tends to be highly specialized, related only to separate parts of her body and not at all to her emotional needs. This can be a very fragmenting experience, nicely described as the alienation of labor. What they do have to offer a laboring woman in distress is not social support but medication. Several recent studies have shown an inverse correlation between these two factors. William Henneborn and Rosemary Cogan found that in all stages of labor, women whose husbands stayed with them throughout labor and delivery experienced less pain and had a lower probablity of receiving medication than women whose husbands stayed with them only in first-stage labor.[124] Another found the husband's support to be an alternative to medication specifically because of his assistance in his wife's breathing and relaxation techniques.[125] The irony of the situation is that the hospital itself creates the stressful conditions under which women require medication to manage their labor.

Another, very recent study of the quality of women's birth experience found that increasing levels of awareness and the husband's participation were both highly related to the enjoyment of the experience.[126] And it is precisely awareness, both mental and physical, that is diminished by analgesia and anesthesia. Mild medication reduces a woman's capacity to be sensitive to the social support of others and to the sensation of giving birth, which many women report to be extremely pleasurable.[127] More medication may eliminate conscious awareness altogether, either by putting the mother to sleep or by causing her to forget everything afterward.

The combination of barring fathers from being present at birth and reducing mothers' consciousness means that the number of people in our society who have actually witnessed a birth is considerably smaller than it used to be, even forty years ago when half of all babies were born at home. It is easy to understand why birth has become such a frightening, mysterious, alien event. Not only is the mother isolated from her family, her friends, and her own body, but she is quickly separated from her new baby as well.

When the baby is born, it is usually shown to the mother and then removed, sometimes for the next twelve or even twenty-four hours.[128] Pioneering research on the effects of this hospital routine has been done by Doctors Marshall Klaus and John Kennell at Case Western Reserve University.[129] Their studies showed that women who had their babies with them immediately after birth and who were allowed five hours of undisturbed contact with their babies in each of the first three days after birth had significantly different behavior patterns than those of a control group of mothers and infants. This group had followed the hospital routine of separation at birth for six to twelve hours, then thirty-minute visits at four-hour intervals for bottle feeding. Observations at one-month examinations of the babies revealed that the longer-contact mothers were more reluctant to leave their infants and engaged in more fondling and soothing behaviors and eye-to-eye contact with the infants. Follow-up studies at one year and three years revealed the same striking differences.

Some hospitals provide mothers the option of rooming-in with their infants, but many still do not. A matched-control-group study in Sweden of first mothers who roomed in with their infants with those who did not revealed that the first group of mothers acquired more competence, self-confidence, and "maternal feelings" and a better understanding of their infants' behavior.[130] So mothers who spend more time with their infants learn how to take care of them more quickly. This early learning is most important with regard to breast-feeding, which tends to be easily discouraged in modern societies.[131] In the hospital Shaw studied, even mothers who intended to breast-feed were separated from their infants for twelve hours after birth.[132]

Klaus and Kennell have also attributed the common condition of postpartum depression to the early separation of mothers and infants and such other hospital practices as the caretaking of the infant by "experts" and the limiting of visitors.[133] Other authors have related postpartum depression directly to the extent of medical intervention in the birth.[134] Estimates are that over 80 percent of mothers experience "postpartum blues" in American hospitals.[135] Now that we no longer have epidemic puerperal fever, postpartum depression is the epidemic maternal iatrogenic disease of the twentieth century.

Thus far we have been looking at the iatrogenic effects of enforced separation on new mothers, but research has shown that the infant is affected as well. In fact, the whole idea of a human attachment depends on a conception of infants, not as passive organisms but as individuals who respond to the people around them.[136] Although it was long assumed that young babies are too immature to appreciate their environment, new research is showing the considerable alertness and awareness of neonates born without the effects of medication.[137] Such infants typically experience a "quiet, alert state" for forty five to sixty minutes after birth, after which they fall into a deep sleep.[138] During this short period, infants will follow a moving object with their eyes, turn their heads to sounds, and bring their hands to their mouths.[139] On the other hand, infants born to mothers who had received analgesia and anesthesia have shown diminished responsiveness to both auditory and visual stimuli.[140] Medication has also been shown to reduce the sucking response, resulting in reduced food intake.[141] For our purposes, the significance of all these effects of maternal medication on the neonate is the reduction of his ability to interact with his environment, particularly his mother and father. Unmedicated mothers and infants will seek eye-to-eye contact with each other, an activity apparently rewarding to both.[142] In fact, infants seem to find the human face the most appealing visual stimulus.[143] But infants who miss this early social interaction because they are sleepy, unresponsive, or simply separated from their mothers may show the effects long after birth. In one study, babies who had experienced both heavy medication and separation were found at thirty and sixty weeks of age to be less interested in social interaction with their mothers and more likely to stimulate themselves with activities such as thumb sucking.[144]

The period after birth should ideally be a time for the newly formed family to get to know each other, to share the rewards of the labor they have all been through. Hospital practices that inhibit family contact weaken these primary social bonds and rob parents and children of one of the richest experiences of human life.

From a sociological point of view, the practice of hospital child-birth constitutes something of an assault on the social relationships of the family—between wives and husbands, parents and children, and siblings. In any way that the hospital unnecessarily prevents family members from being together or from being fully aware of themselves and each other, it handicaps family formation at its inception.

This critique of hospital childbirth is not original to this book. Since the publication of Suzanne Arms's *Immaculate Deception* in 1975, the practice of childbirth in American hospitals has been under attack from all sides—by feminists, members of the counterculture, some elements of the medical profession itself, and ordinary families who did not understand why they could not have a more meaningful experience of the birth of their own children. This critique, at various levels of sophistication, has become public knowledge and is forming the basis for the creation of a whole range of alternatives, from the in-hospital birthing room to do-it-yourself home delivery. The majority of these families are choosing to opt out of the hospital altogether, as we shall see in the next section. Just as animals seek privacy for delivering their young, many young families are seeking safety and intimacy for birth in their own home.

## The Home Birth Movement

There are no hospital costs of any kind to people who have their babies at home. As we have seen, it was not so long ago that the home was the usual place for American babies to be born. In most of the rest of the world, things never changed. Some 98 percent of all the people now alive were born at home, as were the majority of Americans over age sixty. The number of babies being born in American homes today is quite small but apparently growing. The National Center for Health Statistics reports that out-of-hospital births made up only 1.0 percent of total births in 1978, but that represents a small increase over the 1973 figure of 0.7 percent.[145] These figures may also be an underestimation, because data were gathered from birth certificates and some out-of-hospital births may not have been registered. Births that took place on the way to the hospital are counted as hospital births.

Although relatively small in numbers, the home birth movement is widespread and extremely vocal. The publicity it has received may be quite deceptive in this respect. This publicity is largely self-generated by educated, articulate people for whom this is a new and exciting experience. But in reality there appear to be two distinct populations of people who choose to have their babies at home. There is one group for whom the home as the preferred place of birth never changed, whether because of tradition, poverty, or inaccessibility of a hospital. This is still true of many communities, particularly in the rural South[146] and in some ethnic communities in urban areas.[147] Some northern cities historically had midwifery centers that served poor women in their own homes. *The Chicago Maternity Center Story* is a film about one of the oldest of these centers and its recent controversial closing. The moving testimony of the women in this film, who speak of the dignity of having a baby at home and the degradation of delivering in the hospital, should change the mind of anyone who believes that home birth is a middle-class fad.

On the other hand, it is true that growing numbers of home births are taking place among people who were themselves mostly born in hospitals. It is this group that writes the books and makes the films about their experience. Books on home birth are written by mothers and fathers from all regions of the country. There are now at least four national organizations to assist couples planning home births. It is impossible to say whether the trend will continue, but there is some evidence to suggest that it will. In one study of lay midwifery in Texas, 81.8 percent of women who had had experiences with both home and hospital delivery preferred future babies to be born at home.[148] Other studies of such women have found similar results.[149] This indicates that informal, word-of-mouth information on home childbirth will very likely be mainly positive and enthusiastic.

The most complete study of the social characteristics of this new home birth population is an ethnography of 300 home births in the San Francisco Bay area.[150] The couples studied were overwhelmingly middle class; 90 percent lived in single-family dwellings, owned cars, were not on welfare, had some college education, and were employed. The other 10 percent were classified as part of the "hip" culture, meaning they lived communally and considered themselves in rebellion against middle-class values. Another, larger study population from the same area showed some class differences between those couples who engaged lay midwives to help with the birth and those who used physicians.[151] The former group tended to belong more to the counterculture than the other, and the latter included more professional couples. One reason the poor are underrepresented in both groups is that Medicaid in California covers only hospital deliveries, and few getting such help would be able to pay the doctor's or midwife's bill themselves. In rural northern California, one lay midwife's clients are about evenly divided between those on welfare and what she calls the "working poor."[152] Although the self-imposed poverty of the counterculture should probably be distinguished from other urban and rural poverty, there does seem to be a relation between class and the type of birth attendant chosen, with lay midwives more often attending the poor.

There are no clear-cut relationships with religion. Certain religious groups in our society have long-established traditions of midwifery practice, such as the Mormons, Jehovah's Witnesses, Seventh Day Adventists, Hutterites, and Christian Scientists. Many in these groups never gave up having their babies at home. The Farm, a commune in Summertown, Tennessee, is a new "church" that has developed an extensive midwifery practice and a popular book, *Spiritual Midwifery*.[153] The lay midwife in northern California mentioned before estimated that 60 percent of the families she saw had "very strong" religious convictions and tended to express them openly.[154]

The new home birth movement appears to be a primarily white, middle-class phenomenon. With few exceptions, the couples shown in the pictures in the numerous books are white.[155] The study of traditional midwifery in the Houston area, however, found 80 percent of the mothers to be black or Mexican American and only 20 percent Caucasian. The midwives there were all black or Mexican American.[156] At its closing, the Chicago Maternity Center's home birth population was 45 percent black, 40 percent Hispanic, and 15 percent white.[157]

The response of hospitals to the increasing numbers of home births has been predictably negative, as has been that of most of the medical profession. Home birth constitutes a fundamental economic threat to hospitals. Maternity wards are "clean" wards, and hospitals can hardly be expected to want to give them up. Doctors, who are theoretically free to practice in home or hospital, rarely do home deliveries and may even refuse prenatal care to a woman who plans to give birth at home.[158] Physicians and nurses in hospitals often resent families who plan on home births but who rely on the hospital as a backup in case of complications.[159] The negative attitude of many physicians was made explicit in 1976 by the New York chapter of the American College of Obstetricians and Gynecologists, which issued a strong statement opposing any form of out-of-hospital delivery on the grounds that it was unsafe for both mother and child.[160]

Of course there are physicians in many states doing home deliveries. The National Center for Health Statistics data indicate that 11,300, or more than one-third, of the out-of-hospital births in 1975 were attended by physicians.[161] A number of associations formed to promote home childbirth are composed of both enthusiastic professionals and parents. The National Association of Parents and Professionals for Safe Alternatives in Childbirth[162] and the American College of Home Obstetrics[163] were both founded, in part, by concerned physicians. Leading research on the question has been done by medical professionals.[164] And there are some doctors who do quite a few home deliveries.[165] Such doctors learn to develop new skills appropriate to the home situation, especially patience and a hesitancy to intervene in the birth process.

Another recent response of the medical profession to the home childbirth movement has been the growth of alternative birth centers or maternity centers that emphasize natural childbirth and make an attempt to be more homelike. One of the first of these centers was the Childbearing Center of the Maternity Center Association of New York City. Others include the Booth Maternity Center in suburban Philadelphia, the Alternative Birth Center at San Francisco General Hospital, and Lucinia, a birth center in Cottage Grove, Oregon. In all these birth centers, extensive prenatal care, childbirth education, and generally the delivery of the baby are the responsibility of nurse-midwives.[166] But there is some opposition to the idea. *All* out-of-hospital births, including those in birth centers, have been condemned by the American College of Obstetricians and Gynecologists. On the other hand, many parents see the home as the most desirable birthplace. As a midwife at the Childbearing Center commented, "For some people we're too radical. For others we're too institutional." But the idea is growing.

Almost two-thirds of the out-of-hospital births are attended by midwives, only some of whom have formal medical training. The only certification in midwifery granted in the United States is that of certified nurse-midwife, which can be given to registered nurses. But nurse-midwives in many states are licensed to work only in institutions and thus risk their licenses by attending home births. A new group of lay midwives is growing up to meet the new demand for expertise at home births. Many communities have always had such self-trained women, but many have not, particularly the middle-class suburbs where the increase in home births is taking place. Thus a distinctly new group of lay midwives has arisen in the last eight to ten years, some of whom have enjoyed national recognition from their popular books.[167] There are both medical and nonmedical experts to help people have their babies at home, but evidently there are not enough of either as the demand continues to grow. Families who wish to have their babies at home may have to go to great lengths to find someone who will assist them. Some never do find anyone and may decide to go it alone. There is clearly a need here that is not being addressed. Families do have the right to decide where their children will be born. They should certainly also have access to whatever information and assistance they need to carry out the choice they have made.

The issue most often raised with regard to the whole question of home birth, both by those in favor of it and by those against, is the question of safety. As we saw earlier, the major reason for the rapid change to hospitalizing birth during this century was the perception, shared by both the medical profession and families, that the hospital was the safe place to give birth. Undoubtedly there were and are mothers and babies who owe their lives to medical interventions that could only have taken place in hospitals. But the overwhelming majority of all births, 90 to 95 percent, are normal and do not require medical intervention. In addition, the few that present complications are almost always able to be identified long before labor begins. Many parents are convinced that the home is just as safe a place as the hospital for the normal birth, and the few studies done on the subject support this position. Mehl and his colleagues' study of outcomes of 1,146 home births showed fetal and infant death rates considerably below the California state averages and fewer complications of labor and delivery.[168] Mehl's review of home delivery research indicates that all of the few available studies show very favorable outcomes for home deliveries.[169] His own study of two matched populations having home and hospital births showed significantly more birth injuries, resuscitations, and procedures used among hospital births.[170] It must be pointed out that these happy outcomes for home births are primarily the result of careful screening, which is just as it should be. The higher rates of complications, interventions, morbidity, and mortality to some extent reflect the higher risk categories of mothers who chose to go to the hospital. But for low medical risk women, the home appears to be a reasonably safe alternative to hospital birth; indeed, given the possible iatrogenic effect of many of the routine hospital procedures described above, the home may actually be perceived as the safest place to give birth.

The safety of home births is a major factor in many families' decisions to have a home birth, just as it was a major factor in the move to the hospital. People continue to want the best for their children, and their perception of what is best continues to change. The decision to have a home birth is one that is not taken lightly or simply. The reasons people give for their decision are complex and typically well thought out. The literature commonly divides the reasons into categories of medical, psychological, social, and even economic advantages. But their arguments can all be summed up this way: having a child at home is *safer* and *more meaningful*. Given the expectation of a normal delivery, most couples feel that their home is safer than a hospital, both in a physical and in an emotional sense. Because they tend to see pregnancy and childbirth as non-medical life events, they see minimal or no medical intervention as the norm. They do not need the hospital because they are not sick. As one young father commented;

> Hospital birth is like having sex at Masters and Johnson's laboratory. If you have something wrong with your sex life, then you would be grateful to be able to have your sex life dissected. But to have to go there because something *might* go wrong would be crazy.[171]

At home episiotomies, induced or stimulated labor, and medication are not routine and are administered only if necessary. And because the mother is able to move around to find her most comfortable position and eat when she feels like it, childbearing is said to be easier.[172] Many of the couples who advocate home birth are concerned about health; they fill their kitchens with health foods and books on nutrition and are typically concerned about the environment and ecology.[173]

The home is also an emotionally safe place to have a baby. The peaceful familiarity of the surroundings, the privacy, and the quiet make for an environment at once more supportive and more under control. The safety of the home permits an emotional closeness and vulnerability not open to couples in most hospitals even if the husband is permitted to stay with his wife. Home birth represents many things to the people who have done it. But for everyone who has experienced it, it is an event not likely to be forgotten.

Such important events in people's lives are frequently occasions when values are articulated and, not surprisingly, people usually talk about home childbirth as part of some larger belief system. The strong link between home childbirth and traditional (and nontraditional) religious beliefs has already been mentioned. Even among the most secularized parts of our society, though, there is evidence of enthusiasm for home birth, and it fits in well with strong beliefs in feminism, ecology, back-to-nature life-styles, body awareness, and the human potential movement.

Most important, home birth couples seem to share a strong belief in the value of families. Once labor is completed and the baby is born, the baby born at home gets his first introduction into human society:

> In the manner that the mother and father speak to the newborn and in which they touch and hold their child they are communicating (often quite unconsciously) how the world is: whether it is a hostile, frightening place, or secure and loving. It is thus that the infant is introduced to human culture.[174]

It seems somehow most appropriate that the first aspect of our culture a baby should know is its family.

One theme in the literature is that of childbirth as a sacred rite, but there is another theme that is parallel but much more down to earth. In our society the act of having a baby at home is a political act, highlighting questions of power and control. Though men and women do, technically, have the right to decide where and how their baby will be born, laws and policies may prevent them from finding someone competent and willing to help them. The choice of a home birth is not one option among several equal possibilities; it does entail taking control of the situation. In a sense, this is an example of the family seizing control over an act that had become squarely placed in the medical domain and under its control. The woman who gives birth in her own home takes responsibility for the act and its outcome into her own hands. The doctor or midwife comes to her when she calls and is welcomed as her guest. Most couples who have a home birth do have a birth attendant for extra help and expertise, but they do not give over control of the situation or primary responsibility for it. They become conscious, active, and critical participants in the childbirth experience.

Giving birth at home is a phenomenon that almost, but not quite, disappeared from the American scene. The removal of birth from home to hospital unquestionably diminished some of the richness of intimate family life. The attempt in the last few years to bring the experience back into the family reclaims it on somewhat altered terms; unlike the participants in childbirth of the eighteenth, nineteenth, and early twentieth centuries, those present at the birth are more likely to be the nuclear family than the female relatives of the mother. Seeing the birth of their own children is an experience more and more new mothers and fathers are unwilling to give up. In reclaiming childbirth from the hospital's medical control, parents are seeking to demystify medicine and fully experience childbirth for themselves.

## CONCLUSION

Families care *about* themselves, and one of the ways they show that is in caring *for* themselves. Some of these activities are taken so much for granted that they resist our awareness even when we try to think of what families do to care for health. Some are performed automatically and forgotten so quickly that they can be revealed only by a daily health diary. On the other hand, some family health activities are so deliberately undertaken and so exciting that they inspire people to write books about their experience. In between is a range of actions that make use of acquired knowledge, skills, and supplies to promote and protect health, to treat minor illness and injury, and to care for the chronically ill.

What we have tried to emphasize in this chapter is that many of these things have been going on for a long time. Self-care is not a fad. Even home childbirth, which looks at first glance like a radical movement, is in reality simply the reversal of a recent medical trend. Something that is truly new, which we predict will continue to grow in importance, is home care for the chronically ill, a population definitely on the increase. It is the oldness and the newness of the practices in this chapter and the next two that account for the most satisfying aspects of mediating structures, their history and traditions and their creative innovative potential for creating new social forms.

## REFERENCES

1.  Christopher Lasch, *Haven in a Heartless World: The Family Besieged* (New York: Basic Books, 1977).
2.  Talcott Parsons and Renee Fox, "Illness, Therapy, and the Modern Urban American Family," *Journal of Social Issues* 8 (1952): 31–44.
3.  Ibid., p. 43.

4.  Thomas McKeown, *The Role of Medicine: Dream, Mirage or Nemesis?* (London: Nuffield Provincial Hospitals Trust, 1976), p. 94.

5.  Lillian Krueger, "Motherhood on the Wisconsin Frontier, I, II," *Wisconsin Magazine of History* 29 (1945): 157-83, 333–46; R. Carlyle Buley, "Pioneer Health and Medical Practices in the Old Northwest Prior to 1840," *Mississippi Valley Historical Review* 20 (1934): 497-520.

6.  Richard H. Shryock, *Medicine and Society in America, 1660-1860,* (New York: New York University Press, 1960), pp. 95-100.

7.  William G. Rothstein, *American Physicians in the Nineteenth Century: From Sects to Science,* (Baltimore: Johns Hopkins University Press, 1972), part II; Shryock, *Medicine and Society in America.*

8.  Rothstein, *American Physicians in the Nineteenth Century,* ch. 7; Shryock, *Medicine and Society in America,* pp. 145, 171; Ronald L. Numbers, "Do-It-Yourself the Sectarian Way," in Guenter Risse, Ronald L. Numbers, and Judith Walzer Leavitt, eds., *Medicine without Doctors: Home Health Care in American History* (New York: Science History Publications, 1977), pp. 49–72.

9.  Thomson, quoted in Rothstein, *American Physicians in the Nineteenth Century,* p. 139.

10. Ibid., chap. 8.

11. Ibid.

12. Risse, Numbers, and Leavitt, eds., *Medicine without Doctors,* p. 58.

13. John B. Blake, "From Buchan to Fishbein: The Literature of Domestic Medicine," in Risse, Numbers, and Leavitt, eds., *Medicine without Doctors,* pp. 11-30.

14. Ibid.

15. Regina Morantz, "The Lady and Her Physician," in Mary Hartman and Lois Banner, eds., *Clio's Consciousness Raised* (New York: Harper Colophon Books, 1974), pp. 38-53.

16. Regina Markell Morantz, "Nineteenth-Century Health Reform and Women: A Program of Self-Help," in Risse, Numbers, and Leavitt, eds., *Medicine without Doctors,* pp. 73-94.

17. Carroll Smith-Rosenberg, "The Female World of Love and Ritual: Relations between Women in Nineteenth-Century America," *Signs* 1 (1975): 1-29.

18. Rothstein, *American Physicians in the Nineteenth Century,* p. 279.

19. John B. McKinlay and Sonja M. McKinlay, "The Questionable Contribution of Medical Measures to the Decline of Mortality in the United States in the Twentieth Century," *Health and Society* 55 (1977): 405-28.

20. Lasch, *Haven in a Heartless World,* chaps. 5, 6.

21. Ann Douglas Wood, "'The Fashionable Diseases': Women's Complaints and Their Treatment in Nineteenth Century America," in Hartman and

Banner, eds., *Clio's Consciousness Raised*, pp. 1-22; Barbara Ehrenreich and Dierdre English, "Complaints and Disorders: The Sexual Politics of Sickness" (New York: Feminist Press, 1973).

22.  G.J. Barker-Benfield, *The Horrors of the Half-Known Life: Male Attitudes toward Women and Sexuality in Nineteenth-Century America* (New York: Harper & Row, 1976).

23.  Elizabeth M. Whalen, *A Baby?—Maybe* (New York: Bobbs-Merrill, 1975).

24.  Marshall H. Klaus and John H. Kennell, *Maternal-Infant Bonding: The Impact of Early Separation or Loss on Family Development* (St. Louis: C.V. Mosby, 1976).

25.  Thomas Gordon, *Parent Effectiveness Training: The Tested New Way to Raise Responsible Children* (New York: David McKay, 1970).

26.  Ann Oakley, *The Sociology of Housework* (New York: Random House, 1974).

27.  Donald M. Vickery and James F. Fries, *Take Care of Yourself* (Reading, Mass.: Addison-Wesley, 1976).

28.  Ivan Illich, *Medical Nemesis: The Expropriation of Health* (London: Marion Boyars, 1975), p. 165.

29.  Lester Breslow, "A Quantitative Approach to the World Health Organization Definition of Health," *International Journal of Epidemiology* 1, no. 4 (Winter 1972): 347–55; N.B. Belloc and L. Breslow, "Relationship of Physical Health Status and Health Practices," *Preventive Medicine* 1, no. 3 (August 1972): 409–21.

30.  National Analysts, Inc., *A Study of Health Practices and Opinions* (Springfield, Va.: National Technical Information Service, United States Department of Commerce, June 1972).

31.  C.D. Williams, "Health Begins at Home: Reflections on the Theme of W.H.O. Day, 1973," *Journal of Tropical Medicine* 76, no. 7 (1973): 210.

32.  Theodor J. Litman, "The Family as a Basic Unit in Health and Medical Care: A Social Behavioral Overview," *Social Science and Medicine* 5 (1974): 495–519.

33.  E.L. Koos, *The Health of Regionville* (New York: Columbia University Press, 1954).

34.  I.M. Rosenstock, "What Research in Motivation Suggests for Public Health," *American Journal of Public Health* 50, no. 3 (March 1960): 295–301.

35.  David Landy, *Culture, Disease, and Healing: Studies in Medical Anthropology* (New York: Macmillan, 1977).

36.  Peter K. Manning and Horacio Fabrega, "The Experience of Self and Body: Health and Illness in the Chiapas Highlands," in George Psathas, ed., *Phenomenological Sociology* (New York: John Wiley and Sons, 1973), pp. 251–301.

37.  Lois Pratt, *Family Structure and Effective Health Behavior: The Energized Family* (Boston: Houghton Mifflin, 1976).

38.  Irving K. Zola, "Healthism and Disabling Medicalization," in Ivan Illich, *Disabling Professions,* pp. 41–67.

39.  René Dubos, "Health and Creative Adaptation," *Human Nature* 1 no. 1 (January 1978): 74–82.

40.  L. Schneiderman, "Social Class, Diagnosis, and Treatment," *American Journal of Orthopsychiatry* 35 (January 1965): 99–105.

41.  R. Ryan Haynes, D. Wayne Taylor, and David L. Sackett, eds., *Compliance in Health Care* (Baltimore: Johns Hopkins University Press, 1979).

42.  John Fry and the Panel on Self Care, "Self Care: Its Place in the Total Health Care System," 1973, mimeo. p. 8.

43.  Ibid., p. 10.

44.  Ibid., p. 12.

45.  Kerr L. White et al., "International Comparisons of Medical-Care Utilization," *New England Journal of Medicine* 277 (1961): 5106–22.

46.  Litman, "Family as a Basic Unit"; Pratt, *Family Structure.*

47.  Klaus J. Roghmann and Robert J. Haggerty, "The Diary as a Research Instrument in the Study of Health and Illness Behavior: Experiences with a Random Sample of Young Families," *Medical Care* 10, no. 2 (March–April 1972): 143–63.

48.  Fry, "Self Care," p. 8.

49.  *FDA Study* (National Analysts, Inc.), 1972, U.S. Department of Commerce, p. i.

50.  Lois Pratt, "The Significance of the Family in Medication," *Journal of Comparative Family Studies* 4, no. 1 (Spring 1973): 13–32.

51.  Karen Dunnell and Ann Cartwright, *Medicine Takers, Prescribers and Hoarders* (London: Routledge and Kegan Paul, 1972).

52.  David A. Knapp and Deanne E. Knapp, "Decision-Making and Self-Medication: Preliminary Findings," *American Journal of Hospital Pharmacy* 29, no. 12 (1972): 1004–12.

53.  Ibid., p. 1007.

54.  Ibid., p. 1010.

55.  Stella R. Quah, "Self-Medication: A Neglected Dimension of Health Behavior," *Sociological Symposium* no. 19 (1977): p. 27.

56.  C.P. Elliot-Binns, "An Analysis of Lay Medicine," *Journal of the Royal College of General Practitioners* (April 1973): 255–64.

57.  Paol Pederson, "Varighed fra sygdoms begyndelse til praktiserende laege," *Ugeskr Lasfg* 138, no. 32 (August 2, 1976): 1962–66.

58.  John D. Williamson and Kate Danaher, *Self-Care in Health* (London: Croom Helm, 1978), p. 54.

59.    Pearl S. German, "Characteristics and Health Behavior of the Aged Population," *The Gerontologist* (August 1975).

60.    Richard H. Grant, "Family and Self-Help Education in Isolated Rural Communities," in Arlene Fonaroff and Lowell S. Levin, eds., "Issues in Self-Care," *Health Education Monographs*, vol. 5, no. 2 (Summer 1977), pp. 145–60.

61.    Ian I. Findlay, et al., "Chronic Disease in Childhood: A Study of Family Reactions," *British Journal of Medical Education* 3 (1969).

62.    See annotated bibliography in Lowell S. Levin, Alfred H. Katz, and Erik Holst, *Self-Care: Lay Initiatives in Health*, 2d ed. (New York: Prodist, 1979).

63.    Lawrence L. Weed, *Medical Records, Medical Education and Patient Care* (Cleveland: The Press of Case Western Reserve, 1969).

64.    Ruth W. Page, in Weed, *Medical Records,* p. 2.

65.    With regard to the self-care capabilities of children, see Peter Levine, "Efficacy of Self-Therapy in Hemophilia" *New England Journal of Medicine* 291 (1974): 381; M.H. Williams and C. Shim, *Asthma: Discussions in Patient Management* (Flushing, N.Y.: Medical Examination, 1976): pp. 78-79.

66.    Eleanor Anderson, Thomas P. Anderson, and Frederic J. Kotke, "Stroke Rehabilitation: Maintenance of Achieved Gains," *Archives of Physical Medicine and Rehabilitation* 58 (August 1977): 353.

67.    David Agle, "Psychological Factors in Hemophilia: The Concept of Self-Care," *Annals of the New York Academy of Sciences* 240 (1975): 221-25.

68.    Margaret Read, *Culture, Health and Disease* (Philadelphia: Lippincott, 1966).

69.    Ruth Gale Elder, "Social Class and Lay Explanations of the Etiology of Arthritis," *Journal of Health and Social Behavior* 14 (March 1973): 28-38.

70.    Marlene Mackie, "Lay Perceptions of Heart Disease in an Alberta Community," *Canadian Journal of Public Health* 64 (September–October 1973): 445-54.

71.    V.A. Christopherson, "Family Reactions to Illness," in *Living in the Multigenerational Family* (Institute of Gerontology, University of Michigan, 1969), pp. 75-82.

72.    Pratt, *Family Structure.*

73.    Litman, "Family as a Basic Unit," p. 509.

74.    American Hospital Association, *Report of a Conference on Care of Chronically Ill Adults*, Chicago, 1971.

75.    See reference to the work of Bursten and D'Esopo in Stanislav V. Kasl and Sidney Cobb, "Health Behavior, Illness Behavior, and Sick-Role

Behavior," *Archives of Environmental Health* 12 (April 1966): 537.

76.  Margaret M. Jacobson and Robert L. Eichorn, "How Families Cope with Heart Disease: A Study of Problems and Resources," *Journal of Marriage and the Family* (May 1964): 166–73.

77.  Lois Pratt, "Conjugal Organization and Health," *Journal of Marriage and the Family* (February 1972): 85–95.

78.  Richard Wertz and Dorothy C. Wertz, *Lying-In: A History of Childbirth in America* (New York: Free Press, 1977), chap. 1.

79.  Frances E. Kobrin, "The American Midwife Controversy: A Crisis of Professionalization," *Bulletin of the History of Medicine,* 40 (1966): 350–63.

80.  Rosemary Stevens, *American Medicine and the Public Interest* (New Haven, Conn.: Yale University Press, 1971), pp. 99–100.

81.  Neal Devitt, "The Transition from Home to Hospital Birth in the United States, 1930–1960," *Birth and the Family Journal* 4 (1977): 47–58.

82.  National Center for Health Statistics, *Final Natality Statistics, 1978,* DHHS Publication No. (PHS) 80–1120, vol. 29, no. 1, supplement, April 28, 1980.

83.  Wertz and Wertz, *Lying-In,* pp. 148–54.

84.  Ibid., p. 133.

85.  Ibid., p. 155.

86.  Devitt, "Transition from Home to Hospital Birth," p. 56.

87.  "A Place to be Born," *British Medical Journal,* January 10, 1976, p. 55.

88.  Devitt, "Transition from Home to Hospital Birth," p. 56.

89.  Wertz and Wertz, *Lying-In,* pp. 148–50.

90.  Victor R. Fuchs, *Who Shall Live?* (New York: Basic Books, 1974), p. 60.

91.  Michael Whitt, M.D., quoted in Suzanne Arms, *Immaculate Deception* (New York: Bantam Books, 1977), p. 64.

92.  New York Academy of Medicine, *Maternal Mortality in New York City* (New York: Commonwealth Fund, 1933).

93.  White House Conference on Child Health and Family Protection, *Fetal, Newborn, and Maternal Mortality and Morbidity* (New York, 1933), pp. 215–17.

94.  A.L. Cochrane, *Effectiveness and Efficiency* (London: Nuffield Provincial Hospitals Trust, 1972), p. 63.

95.  Ibid., p. 64.

96.  Devitt, "Transition from Home to Hospital Birth," p. 57.

97.  Quoted in Arms, *Immaculate Deception,* p. 44.

98.  Statistical Office of the United Nations, *Demographic Yearbook, 1977,* pp. 332–35.

99.  Summarized in Arms, *Immaculate Deception,* pp. 51–57.

100.  Rebecca Rowe Parfitt, *The Birth Primer* (Philadelphia: Running Press, 1977), p. 69.

101.  Arms, *Immaculate Deception,* p. 65.
102.  Devitt, "Transition from Home to Hospital Birth," p. 51.
103.  Wertz and Wertz, *Lying-In,* p. 242.
104.  M.P.M. Richards, "Innovation in Medical Practice: Obstetricians and the Induction of Labour in Britain," *Social Science and Medicine,* 9 (1975): 595–602.
105.  Arms, *Immaculate Deception,* p. 111.
106.  Nancy Stoller Shaw, *Forced Labor: Maternity Care in the United States* (New York: Pergamon Press, 1974), p. 67.
107.  Roberto Caldeyro-Barcia, "Some Consequences of Obstetrical Interference," *Birth and the Family Journal* 2 (1975): 34–38, 73–76.
108.  Lewis Mehl et al., "Home vs. Hospital Birth: A Matched Comparison Study," (paper presented at American Public Health Association, Miami, Florida, 1976).
109.  Quoted in Frederic M. Ettner, "Comparative Study of Obstetrics," in *Safe Alternatives in Childbirth* 3d ed., David Stewart and Lee Stewart, eds., Safe Alternatives in Childbirth (Chapel Hill, N.C.: National Association of Parents and Professionals for Safe Alternatives in Childbirth, 1978), pp. 41–42.
110.  Doris Haire, *The Cultural Warping of Childbirth* (Milwaukee: International Childbirth Education Association, 1972).
111.  Arms, *Immaculate Deception,* p. 111.
112.  Ibid., p. 101.
113.  Malca Aleksandrowicz, "The Effect of Pain Relieving Drugs Administered during Labor and Delivery on the Behavior of the Newborn: A Review," *Merrill-Palmer Quarterly* 20 (1974): 121–41.
114.  Ibid., pp. 128–29.
115.  Ibid., p. 131.
116.  Ibid., pp. 133–35.
117.  Mehl et al., "Home Vs. Hospital Birth."
118.  Ruth Watson Lubic, "The Effect of Cost on Patterns of Maternity Care," *Nursing Clinics of North America* 10 (1975): 229–39.
119.  Lewis E. Mehl et al., "Outcomes of Elective Home Births: A Series of 1,146 Cases," *Journal of Reproductive Medicine* 19 (1977): 281–90.
120.  Wertz and Wertz, *Lying-In,* p. 4.
121.  Margaret Mead, quoted in Arms, *Immaculate Deception,* pp. 96–97.
122.  Marion Sousa, *Childbirth at Home* (New York: Bantam Books, 1977), p. 7.
123.  Quoted in Lester Dessez Hazell, *Commonsense Childbirth* (New York: Berkley Medallion Books, 1976), p. 122.
124.  William J. Henneborn and Rosemary Cogan, "The Effect of Husband Participation on Reported Pain and Probability of Medication During Labor and Birth," *Journal of Psychosomatic Research* 19 (1975): 215–22.

125.    Kathleen L. Norr et al., "Explaining Pain and Enjoyment in Childbirth," *Journal of Health and Social Behavior* 18 (1977): 260-75.

126.    Susan G. Doering, Doris Entwisle, and Daniel Quinlan, "Modelling the Quality of Women's Birth Experience," *Journal of Health and Social Behavior* 21 (1980): 12-21.

127.    Sheila Kitzinger, *The Experience of Childbirth* (New York: Penguin Books, 1978), pp. 237-40.

128.    Shaw, *Forced Labor*, p. 97.

129.    Marshall H. Klaus and John H. Kennell, *Maternal-Infant Bonding: The Impact of Early Separation or Loss on Family Development* (St. Louis: C.V. Mosby, 1976).

130.    M. Greenberg, I. Rosenberg, J. Lind, "First Mothers Rooming-in with Their Newborns: Its Impact on the Mother," *American Journal of Orthopsychiatry* 43 (1973): 783-88.

131.    Jane Hubert, "Belief and Reality: Social Factors in Pregnancy and Childbirth," in Martin P.M. Richards, ed., *The Integration of a Child into a Social World* (London: Cambridge University Press, 1974), pp. 37-52.

132.    Shaw, *Forced Labor*, p. 97.

133.    Klaus and Kennell, *Maternal-Infant Bonding*, pp. 93-94.

134.    Ann Oakley, *Women Confined: Towards a Sociology of Childbirth* (New York: Schocken, 1980).

135.    Klaus and Kennell, *Maternal-Infant Bonding*, pp. 93-94.

136.    Michael Lewis and Leonard A. Rosenblum, eds., *The Effect of the Infant on Its Caregiver* (New York: John Wiley, 1974).

137.    Frederic Leboyer, *Birth without Violence* (New York: Alfred Knopf, 1975).

138.    Klaus and Kennell, *Maternal-Infant Bonding*, p. 66.

139.    T. Berry Brazelton, "The Early Mother-Infant Adjustment," *Pediatrics* 32 (1963): 931-38.

140.    Aleksandrowicz, "The Effect of Pain Relieving Drugs," p. 135.

141.    Martin Richards, "The One-Day-Old Deprived Child," *New Scientist* 28 (1974): 820-22.

142.    Klaus and Kennell, *Maternal-Infant Bonding*, pp. 70-71.

143.    Ibid.

144.    Richards, "One-Day-Old Deprived Child," p. 821.

145.    National Center for Health Statistics, *Final Natality Statistics, 1978*.

146.    Eliot Wigginton, ed., *Foxfire 2* (Garden City, N.Y.: Anchor Press, 1963), pp. 274-303.

147.    Florence E. Lee and Jay H. Glasser, "Role of Lay Midwifery in Maternity Care in a Large Metropolitan Area," *Public Health Reports* 89 (1974): 537-44.

148.    Ibid.

149.    W.O. Goldthorp and J. Richman, "Maternal Attitudes to Unintended

Home Confinement," *The Practitioner* 212 (1974): 845–53; E.A. Topliss, "Selection Procedure for Hospital and Domiciliary Confinements" in Gordon McLachlan and Richard Shegog, eds., *In the Beginning* (London: Nuffield Provincial Hospitals Trust, 1970), pp. 59–78.

150. Lester Dessez Hazell, *Birth Goes Home: A Study of Couples Electing Home Birth* (Marble Hill, Mo.: NAPSAC, 1975).

151. Mehl et al., "Outcomes of Elective Home Births," pp. 281–90.

152. Nancy Mills, quoted in Charlotte and Fred Ward, *The Home Birth Book* (Garden City, N.Y.; Doubleday, 1977), p. 50.

153. Ina May Gaskin, *Spiritual Midwifery* (Summertown, Tenn.: Book Publishing Company, 1978).

154. Mills, quoted in Ward, *Home Birth Book,* p. 50.

155. Ibid.

156. Lee and Glasser, Role of Lay Midwifery," p. 539.

157. Parfitt, *The Birth Primer,* p. 168.

158. Alice Gilgoff, *Home Birth,* (New York: Coward, McCann and Geoghegan, 1978), p. 88.

159. Margot Edwards, "Unattended Home Birth," *American Journal of Nursing* 73 (1973): 1332–35.

160. Quoted in Wertz and Wertz, *Lying-In,* p. 237.

161. National Center for Health Statistics, *Final Natality Statistics, 1976.*

162. P.O. Box 267, Marble Hill, Mo. 63764.

163. 2821 Rose Street, Franklin Park, Ill. 60103.

164. Mehl, "Outcomes of Elective Home Births."

165. Arms, *Immaculate Deception,* pp. 244–47; Ward, *Home Birth Book,* pp. 35–42.

166. Eunice K. Ernst and Mabel Forde, "Maternity Care: An Attempt at an Alternative," *Nursing Clinics of North America* 10 (1975): 241–49; Alison Rice and Elaine Carty, "Alternative Birth Centers," *The Canadian Nurse* (November 1977).

167. Raven Lang, *Birth Book* (Palo Alto, California: Science and Behavior Books, 1972); Gaskin, *Spiritual Midwifery.*

168. Mehl et al., "Outcomes of Elective Home Births."

169. Lewis E. Mehl, "Home Delivery Research Today—A Review," *Women and Health* 1 (1976): 3–11.

170. Ibid.

171. Quoted in Hazell, *Commonsense Childbirth,* p. 141.

172. Dorothy Fitzgerald et al., *Home Oriented Maternity Experience: A Comprehensive Guide to Home Birth* (Washington, D.C.: HOME, 1976), pp. 10–18.

173. Hazell, *Birth Goes Home.*

174. Sheila Kitzinger, *The Experience of Childbirth,* 4th ed. (New York: Penguin Books 1978), p. 256.

# 3 RELIGIOUS GROUPS AND HEALING

Religious institutions have played a vital role in our country's history, and despite current assumptions of their imminent demise, they remain by far the largest group of voluntary associations in our society. In fact, as Peter Berger and Richard Neuhaus like to point out, more Americans are in church on any single Sunday morning than the total number of people who attend professional sports events in a whole year.[1] Latest available data show that more than 131 million Americans belong to some 333,000 churches.[2] Interestingly, the most recent Gallup Poll figures (1976) show an increase of 2 percent from 1975 in church attendance in an average week nationwide.[3] This increase comes after a twenty-year period of steady decline in church attendance, from 49 percent in 1955 to 40 percent in 1975, a trend commonly viewed as the beginning of the end of American religion. Charts depicting the decline, however, invariably begin with 1955 or 1958, a convenient twenty-year span that seems to imply that church attendance had been higher still in the preceding decades. In fact the opposite is the case. The decade of the 1950s was simply one in a series of religious revivals in this country's history, and to measure current church attendance against these peak years is necessarily misleading. A longer view reveals a fairly steady increase in the percentage of the total population claiming religious membership, from 43 percent in 1910 to

62.4 percent in 1970, with a peak of 69 percent in 1960.[4] A majority of the American people, 58 percent, currently consider their religious beliefs "very important," and an additional 28 percent call them "fairly important."[5] Americans say they are serious about their religious beliefs, and their actions support this. Further, one might even be safe in predicting that the recent 2 percent increase in church attendance is the first step in a new cycle in keeping with the historical pattern of decline and revival.

Public policy debates on questions of religion and health have tended to settle in three areas, within all of which there are significant controversies. In the area of medical ethics, religion has played a significant role in shaping the debates in medical practice, particularly in the areas of abortion, death and dying, and questions surrounding refusal of medical treatment, and in medical research into genetic engineering and *in vitro* fertilization. A second area of significant public policy discussion is that surrounding the religious sponsorship of medical institutions. Religious organizations have had a long history of establishing and staffing hospitals, nursing homes, and most recently hospices, and of sending medical missions abroad. Another new variation on this theme is the Wholistic Health Center, family-practice medical care facilities located in churches, whose staffs are made up of physicians, pastors, and nurses.[6] A third area of debate has been about national health insurance, for which some church groups have lobbied heavily.[7] But public policy debate in all these areas has had a common denominator: it has all been concerned with medical services provided by professionals. Without downplaying the importance of religion's role in these discussions, there is a need to recognize the *direct* link between religion, health, and healing, which is not mediated through the medical profession. Thus this chapter is concerned with those non-professional, indigenous activities that involve religion and health, which, just as in the family, are so much a part of the world people take for granted that they are hard to see. This chapter describes historical and contemporary religious health and healing activities and provides a close look at a specific activity that has been growing in recent years: faith healing among Catholic Pentecostals.

It should be pointed out that the literature used for research in this chapter on religion and health tends to come from within religious groups, rather than from within the medical profession (not surprisingly) or even from within the social sciences. Healing activities in American churches are so widespread and usually so unsensational that they rarely reach the notice of the wider public. Yet there is a vast religious literature on healing, one that seems to grow by the day. These books, much like those on home child-birth, are written by and for believers. It is true that "for the be-liever, no proof is necessary; for the unbeliever no proof is enough." But neither of these groups of literature can be dismissed as unim-portant on the grounds that they are not objective. This literature constitutes a body of evidence that these practices are real for a large number of people in our society who evidently find them meaningful and significant. On this basis alone, then, they constitute an area of lay health activity worthy of consideration.

## THE HEALING QUALITIES OF RELIGION

The relation between religion and health is complex; some attention has already been given to epidemiological evidence for the role religion plays in buffering the social stress that is at the root of so many of the illnesses people suffer in modern society. Religious groups, like families and other mediating structures, seem to blunt the effects of social stress on the individual by providing a physical and emotional shelter, a place of safety. Regardless of their manifest interest in health (and certainly some religious groups are more concerned with health than others), membership in a religious group per se seems to have a latent effect on the health of religious group members. Moreover, the religious group as a mediating struc-ture possesses certain special attributes relevant to illness; religion has a healing quality all its own.

"Religion is the human enterprise by which a sacred cosmos is established."[8] By this is meant that religion is a way of thinking about the world that includes belief in God or some sense of tran-scendence. Such an interpretation of reality is directly relevant to each of the three widespread conditions of modern society related to social stress: rapid social change, alienation, and anomie. The sacred cosmos, whatever form it may take in a particular religious belief system, is invariably transcendental and eternal. It points beyond this life and beyond this world to some greater reality.

When the social values and symbols of earthly communities are threatened by rapidly changing conditions, they may become inadequate, inappropriate, or irrelevant. But religious symbols define the individual's or the community's relation to a set of values and a tradition that are timeless or, better, that include this time and all others, past and future. Religion provides a view of history within which the past and future can be understood and the confusing present can at the very least be seen as temporary, if not understandable.

The second stressful social condition is alienation, perceived as powerlessness. The seemingly intractable social problems of modern society—meaningless work, widespread poverty and unemployment, political injustice, war, and crime—are experienced on the personal level as powerlessness and may be reacted to with frustration and anger or with hopelessness and despair. Belief in the omnipotence of a deity gives an individual access to a power outside himself, infinitely greater than his own. Belief in divine omniscience expands his own understanding.

Third, anomie is perceived as meaninglessness—of life in general, one's own in particular. Anomie is the condition of the lonely, the isolated, those who lack a strong connection with a larger group. Integration into any group adds to one's personal history the history of the group; it both links up with and expands the personal biography. Membership in families links most people to at most four or five generations other than their own. Belonging to a traditional religious community links one to scores of generations with whom one shares some very important beliefs. Membership in religious groups conveys a certain immortality—regardless of whether or not it includes a belief in an afterlife—the immortality of the group. Religious groups also integrate one into widening circles in the present, beyond one's family, to the neighborhood church, to churches in other cities, and to the Christian, Jewish, or other religious community as a whole.

To understand the potential of all religions for healing, it is helpful to conceive of health and illness as order and disorder. As Carl Jung wrote in 1933:

> During the past thirty years, people from all the civilized countries of the earth have consulted me. I have treated many hundreds of patients. . . . Among all my patients in the second half of life—that is to say, over thirty-

five—there has not been one whose problem in the last resort was not that of finding a religious outlook on life. It is safe to say that every one of them fell ill because he had lost that which the living religions of every age have given to their followers, and none of them has been really healed who did not regain his religious outlook.[9]

But it is not necessary to go as far as Jung did to accept the idea that illness is a disorder for which the order of religious ritual and liturgy can be a comfort. The religious understanding of illness as disorder (and, conversely, of health as wholeness) is based on a sense of profound connectedness between body, mind, and spirit, no one of which can be disturbed without influencing the other two. This ancient view of human health and illness has recently become popular again as the basis for holistic medicine. Illness is seen as the expression of conflicts, of disharmony on any of the three levels. There may be conflicts within an individual between competing sets of values or loyalties, between one individual and another, or between an individual and his spiritual world. The relevance of this view of health for religion is that if it is true that the mind (or spirit) can influence the body in the direction of ill health, and vice versa, as psychosomatic medicine attests, then those same channels of communication must be able to carry positive influence as well. The restoration of the individual's relation to God through prayer, confession, and worship both restores his interior balance and reintegrates him into the religious community. Harmony in one's spiritual relationship is inseparable from harmony in social relationships. And restored harmony in both may have apparent healing effect. Religion cannot be just a private matter; it is a common possession of the group. The religious fellowship functions through its shared symbols, and in supporting these symbols the group supports itself. Moreover, these definitions are not the product of any abstract analysis, they are religion's own self-conscious understandings of health and illness in human beings who have bodies, minds, and souls.[10]

This point bears closer examination. Recent work in the social sciences and medicine has revealed significant differences between doctors and patients in their definitions of health and illness. It has become increasingly clear that lay conceptions of standards of wellness and the causes of disease are quite divergent from the medical model.[11] This has long been obvious to medical workers in nonscientific, traditional cultures where indigenous, often religiously oriented healing systems compete openly with Western medicine. What is recently developing among students of social sciences and medicine is an awareness that these cultural differences are alive in our own society, and not only among urban ethnic minorities. Although much work remains to be done in this field before any conclusions can be drawn, one significant inference can be made simply on the basis of the fact that these differences in conceptions of illness exist. One must conclude that where lay explanations of illness involve social or spiritual as well as, or even instead of, purely physical disturbances, real healing must also be social or spiritual. Lay interpretations of illness tend to be highly social, serving to explain individual illness in terms of the relations within the group.[12]

Arthur Kleinman has delineated two "interpenetrating processes" making up healing in traditional systems, which seem to be equally applicable to healing in modern societies. These processes, which are mutually dependent, are the provision of meaning for the experience of illness and attempts to control illness by curing the disease or relieving its symptoms.[13] Kleinman's point is that, whereas in traditional healing these two processes are inseparable, even indistinguishable at times, in modern medical systems efforts to control illness and to provide meaning for it have been divorced. What current critiques are calling the "dehumanization" of medicine is in large measure this abdication of responsibility for providing meaning for the experience of illness. The whole question whether medicine should or even can be expected to provide this meaning is an interesting but thorny problem that, in a way, underlies this entire book. We will not attempt to answer it here. The point to be made is that if healing necessarily involves both the control of illness and the provision of meaning for it and if medicine is not able to provide that meaning, then it must come from some other source if people are to experience real healing.

Another helpful concept in discussions of religion and healing is that of the "assumptive world," a term that refers to the whole complex structure of values, expectations, and knowledge about the world.[14] The assumptive world is *assumed*, meaning that very little of it is in conscious awareness. It underlies human experience and structures the way the world is perceived. Illness is a disturbance in human experience that brings the assumptive world to light; it is a challenge that brings the order into question. Jerome Frank asserts that healing is promoted by consistency of the assumptive worlds of the sick person, the healer, and the social group of which they are a part. Such a convergence of values and beliefs permits much to go unspoken without being misunderstood. Available empirical evidence bears out the importance of convergent assumptive worlds for healing; moreover, it seems as if people even seek out healers on the basis of these assumptions. A study of different medical and nonmedical healing resources in a Malay village revealed that the choice of a healer depended, more than anything else, on the sick person's own interpretation of the cause of his illness. These choices appeared to be highly rational. Native healers were known to have greater success rates with certain disorders than medical therapists, although medical therapy succeeded in other cases. Overall, the success rates of the two were quite comparable.[15] Kleinman notes that in cases where patients' reported improvement is greater after contact with nonmedical healers, the difference can usually be ascribed to small social class differences and a greater concordance of explanatory systems between patient and healer.[16] Assumptive worlds do make a difference—in how people interpret the causes of their illness, in how they choose healers, and in the criteria by which they judge the effectiveness of their healing.

The role of religion in structuring assumptive worlds is important in any case but absolutely critical when it comes to healing. Healing that takes place in a religious context calls into play not only the strength of the social group but also the power of the transcendental. Religious healing always involves ceremonies and rituals that make religious symbols concrete. The beliefs embodied in the ritual help the patient organize the chaos of his illness; they give him a plan of action to cope with it, and they provide a very real, effective way of resolving the conflicts that may lie at the source of the illness. Many religious healing rituals entail a review of the sick person's life, especially as it relates to the current illness, and frequently include confession and forgiveness. In this way past and current events are organized around the condition of the illness, bringing to conscious awareness many social, emotional, or spiritual relationships that had not previously been acknowledged. Thus religious healing exhibits both of Kleinman's processes of healing; it can act to control illness by resolving root conflicts, and it can provide meaning for the experience.

For the student of religious healing, then, it is not necessary to share the faith of the believers to accept the validity of their reports of healing. Such reports must be accepted, knowing that the grounds on which judgments are made will include more than the individual's physical condition. It would also not be wise to explain religious healing purely in terms of psychotherapeutic dynamics, as many writers have done. Medical belief systems and religious belief systems are parallel, alternative ways of interpreting experiences. The latter is not reducible to the former. Thus religious healing cannot be "explained" in terms of suggestion; it has its own reality. Although this realization has come only recently to social scientists,[17] it is a point that theologians have long been making.[18] In fact, it is a common observation among religious writers that God does not reject the instrumentation of natural powers of healing, since he is the author of these as well.[19]

The meanings different religions provide for illnesses vary as much as the religions do. Some faiths value bodily health far more than others do. To some it may be almost completely peripheral. But all faiths offer something that medicine, even at its most humanistic, cannot convey. The end point of medical healing is restoration of the individual to physical or mental health. Some forms of the new holistic medicine broaden this goal considerably to reincorporating the individual within the social group. But the marginal situation of illness does not always end in the restoration of health, no matter how broadly it may be conceived. The ultimate threat to our existence is not illness but death, from which no medicine can finally save us.

All religions *account for* illness, suffering, and death. They place these universal aspects of human biography into a larger context, making them meaningful and bearable. Human consciousness and suffering are uniquely related; neither is possible without the other. A certain level of consciousness is necessary before suffering can be said to exist, and suffering can either enhance or diminish consciousness. Because of these relationships, as Bakan points out, there are two natural options for coping with human suffering.[20] Consciousness may either be obliterated or enhanced through understanding. Medicine can offer relief from suffering through physical or chemical means, and it can also offer a somewhat limited form of understanding by discovering and naming the forms of tissue damage that have led to a particular pain. But only religion can offer understanding in the face of unrelieved suffering and inevitable death.

Such explanations are a part of any religion whose idea of God includes an ethical sense. Max Weber first called these explanations theodicies and recognized them as solutions to the problem of evil and suffering in the world.[21] Religions whose God is a good and just God are left with the fact of human suffering. If God is all-powerful and all-loving, why would he not eliminate evil, pain, and death from the world? The major religious traditions in Western society have addressed this paradox in various ways.

For the Jewish people, God is righteous and just and, because He is omnipotent, all disease and health are seen as morally and spiritually conditioned. Sickness is both a means of punishment for individual or community sin and a means of atonement for guilt. For the Jews, disease and suffering are one of the ways God works in the world to bring about repentance and redemption. Suffering is never purposeless.[22]

Christianity, in addition to its healing tradition has also provided meaning for pain through the preeminent symbol of suffering, the cross. Christians believe that the crucifixion of Jesus Christ shows human beings how to find redemption in their own suffering and a way to overcome the loneliness and privacy of pain. Even if the Christian does not experience physical healing through his faith (which some apparently do), the belief in a God who also suffered, died, and was resurrected clearly places the individual's experience of pain and suffering in a larger, highly meaningful context. Christians and Jews may suffer pain, but they do not suffer meaninglessness. Ernest Becker's brilliant book *The Denial of Death* argues just this point with a remarkable synthesis of psychology and philosophy. He writes:

> One goes through it all to arrive at faith, the faith that one's very creature-liness has some meaning to a Creator; that despite one's true insignificance, weakness, death, one's existence has meaning in some ultimate sense because it exists within an external and infinite scheme of things brought about and maintained to some kind of design by some creative force.[23]

When one links oneself with a transcendental God, one gains some measure of immortality.

The relevance of this insight for an analysis of mediating structures is that only human beings can mediate meaning, even the meaning of the transcendent. Religion is far more than the abstract beliefs of isolated individuals in some transcendent reality. Human beings express their experience of transcendent reality on earth through symbols and rituals, and they most commonly carry out these expressions in groups. Religious activities are stimulating group experiences, which, through the ritualistic means of worship, prayer, and liturgy, seek to bring a close association between symbol and reality. The bonds formed by such sharing are the basis of membership in the religious community. As a mediating structure, then, a religious group provides structure and meaning for individual life and promotes identification with what are really two forms of transcendence: the social and the spiritual. Membership in a religious group overcomes suffering and death by making them meaningful. Certain religious beliefs may gain one the immortality of one's soul, but all shared faiths gain one the immortality of the group of believers.

Religion thus becomes relevant to the problem of illness in two ways. Its healing potential can restore people to health and wholeness or ease them into death. It *is* necessary for an observer to know what is meant by healing because definitions and criteria tend to be specific to different religious groups. It can be generalized, however, that all religious understandings of healing will be broader than medical definitions. They may be quite different both from medical definitions and from those within other religious traditions. Religion is the business of establishing a sacred cosmos. The place and importance of the human body within that sacred cosmos is very different in, say, Seventh Day Adventism and Roman Catholicism, not to mention Presbyterianism and Buddhism. Of the major world religions, healing has had a most important place in Christian history and tradition.

## HEALING AND CHRISTIANITY

### Healing in the Christian Tradition

Early Christianity was, among other things, a healing cult. But healing as a religious practice was a radical break from the Judaic tradition. Physical sickness plays an important role in the Old Testament, and its religious meaning is primarily a break in man's relationship with God. But for the ancient Jews this relationship was not an individual man-God relationship; neither was sickness seen as the affliction of single individuals. In the Old Testament, the stress is on the fate of the group, not that of individuals within it. Thus sickness inflicted by God often came in the form of plagues, from which the whole community suffered.[24]

There was a tradition of healing associated with the Greek temples of Aesculapius, another culture in the ancient world with which the early Christians had some contact. The practice of healing in the Greek temples was called incubation, which involved sleeping in the temple.[25]

Jesus' healing was a centrally important characteristic of his ministry and the early church. In Greek and Aramaic, the words for healing, health, wholeness, and salvation are identical, or nearly so, which would indicate a close connection among these things in Jesus' mind.[26] The New Testament, especially the chapters of Mark, Luke, and Matthew, record no less than forty-one separate healing miracles, making healing a centrally important part of Jesus' ministry. It appears that Jesus' healing was sacramental; that is, it involved the largely symbolic actions of touching with the hands and speaking words. Some healings also occurred when people touched Jesus or even his clothes, as in the case of the woman who suffered from continuous bleeding. The gospels record healings of quite a large variety of illnesses, including both mental and physical ailments, such as leprosy, deafness, blindness, and possession by demons.

If the healing miracles of Jesus' ministry were limited to his earthly lifetime, they would have a purely symbolic meaning for Christians. But the basis of contemporary Christian belief in the power of God's love to heal physical and mental illness today is the record in the New Testament that Jesus sent out his twelve disciples to heal in his name. Healing was intended as an example of the way Christian people were to treat one another. The ability to heal was the true test of an apostle of Jesus, and it continued to be an extremely important part of the life of the early church after Jesus' crucifixion. The classic healing text in the New Testament is part of a letter by the apostle James, written at about the end of the first century:

> Is any among you sick? Let him call for the elders of the church, and let
> them pray over him, anointing him with oil in the name of the Lord; and

the prayer of faith will save the sick man, and the Lord will raise him up; and if he has committed sins he will be forgiven. Therefore confess your sins to one another, and pray for one another, that you may be healed.[27]

The healing ministry of the early Christians was one means of winning new believers. It certainly marked them as different from other contemporary religious groups. Healing was a part of the reality of being a Christian; it was one aspect of the religious experience. So many early Christians received healing, judging from the New Testament and the writings of the early church fathers, that for three centuries the early Christians could take their ability to heal almost for granted. One writer has called it "the expectation of every Christian."[28]

The tradition of healing in the Christian Church did not continue for long at this level of importance, however. The practice of healing in the first few centuries of the life of the church was a continuation of the acts of Jesus and his disciples. The important turning point for these attitudes and practices was the conversion of the emperor Constantine in the fourth century and the radical changes that brought about in a religion that had been that of a persecuted minority. Under Constantine many were forced into conversion whose knowledge and beliefs were hardly held with great conviction. The institutionalization that made Christianity safe for Christians numbed the zeal of the religious experience.[29]

The effective elimination of the healing ministry from the Christian Church for the next fifteen centuries rested on a set of popular and theological beliefs that tended to devalue life on earth and the body that life took place in. After the fall of the Roman Empire, theological thinking shifted from the world view of Plato to that of Aristotle, an increasingly rationalistic view, which Kelsey says left little room for direct healing contact between God and man.[30] But as the body and its healing became less important, the soul and its life after death became more so. The meaning of healing in the Christian tradition, then, did not so much die out as shift quite radically in emphasis, from the healing of the body in this life to the healing of the soul for the next.

The most graphic illustration of this shift is the change in the ritual of anointing for healing.[31] Anointing the sick with oil was an ancient custom adopted by the early Christians, as mentioned in the foregoing passage from the New Testament. Anointing, or unction, could be carried out both by priests and by lay people who had had the olive oil blessed by a priest. The rite was attended by members of the family and the congregation and accompanied by prayers, blessings, and the laying on of hands. But gradually the rite came to be performed with less and less expectation of physical cure, and increasing emphasis was laid on its function of absolving the sick person from sin and saving his soul. By the eleventh or twelfth century, church records show that anointing for healing had become a ritual to assure the dying person that his sins had been forgiven. Unction for healing became extreme unction, and church doctrine required that it be performed at the point of death, to secure a spiritual advantage in the next world.[32]

There was one tradition of religious healing that did continue through the Middle Ages, though its origins were more Greek than Christian. The healing temples of Aesculapius in Greece became Christian healing shrines. Other Christian churches were also believed to have healing power, especially those associated with saints who specialized in miraculous cures or monastic orders that specialized in nursing.[33] The roots of modern hospitals have been traced to this use of Christian churches as shelters for the sick.[34]

Christian tradition, by and large, however, has tended to downplay its own ministry of healing the sick despite the centrality of healing in the New Testament. Without denying that Jesus and his disciples did heal the sick, recent Christian interpretation of these works has seen them as limited to that period of history, a view known as dispensationalism. The argument is that the healing miracles did indeed happen, because God used such works to get his Church established. But because they are no longer necessary, they are no longer possible.[35] Christians, most particularly Protestants, have tended to view suffering in all forms, including sickness, as redemptive. Some theologians have even seen illness as serving God's purpose in bringing forth sympathy, unselfishness, and love in those who care for the sick.[36]

But there has been a perceptible change in the Church's attitude toward healing in the past thirty years, a change that began outside the mainstream Protestant and Catholic churches. This resurgence of interest in healing is a fascinating phenomenon that can best be seen as simply one part of a larger religious revival.

Of course it would be a mistake to imply that all forms of Christian healing had ceased before the current healing revival. Healing shrines have always existed in the Roman Catholic Church and are still the objects of long pilgrimages today. The most famous modern shrine is at Lourdes, in the south of France. Since the mid-nineteenth century, the site has been visited by several million seriously ill people, and innumerable claims of cures have been made. The Catholic Church maintains a rigorously scientific medical bureau at the shrine, which examines all those claiming a cure. It has certified only approximately fifty cases as genuine miracles, rejecting many cures that apparently satisfied the sufferer.[37]

The New Thought and Christian Science movements also began in the nineteenth century and have continued to grow. Mary Baker Eddy founded Christian Science in 1879 as a church that would reject the idea of illness and even the reality of the body. The subsequent success of the church must be attributed to the fact that people found in Christian Science something utterly lacking in other churches of the day.[38]

Healing has also been an integral part of the beliefs of the Pentecostal churches, which began in this country at the turn of the century. The experiences of baptism in the Holy Spirit and glossolalia, or speaking in tongues, began to occur to a group of people in Kansas who recognized them as similar to the New Testament accounts of the disciples' experiences after the crucifixion and resurrection of Christ, the period called Pentecost. The early leaders soon found that healings occurred when converts were baptized and spoke in tongues. Healing, then, was not the center of Pentecostal beliefs but simply one among numerous biblical gifts of the Holy Spirit. The Pentecostal churches, some of the best known of which are the Assemblies of God, the Church of God, and the Pentecostal Holiness churches, have spread across the country, though they have been especially successful in the South. Pentecostal churches claim some 2 million members in this country, and 12 to 15 million followers worldwide.[39]

The growth of Pentecostalism from the beginning of the century to the end of World War II was steady and strong, but the Pentecostal revival that occurred in the postwar period dwarfed this early growth. Moreover, the Pentecostal revival of the late 1940s and 1950s was fundamentally a healing revival.[40] The period was marked by the ecstatic tent revival meetings of traveling evangelists, very much in the tradition of the religious revivals of earlier periods of American history. What was somewhat new was the emphasis on healing and the claims of miracles, as well as the use of radio and eventually television. All the revivalists were careful to claim that healing came only from God, but as God's anointed ministers, they did believe themselves to be essential catalysts in the healing process. Thus there was a good bit of drama and showmanship in the meetings, which marked them as different from the mainstream Protestant services of the day. There were innumerable tent revival ministers, most of whose names would be familiar to few. But the most successful healing revivalists acquired a national reputation, and some, like Oral Roberts and the late Kathryn Kuhlman, continued their ministries, albeit with some changes, well into the 1970s.

Kathryn Kuhlman and Oral Roberts were hardly the only evangelist-healers during this period, though they were arguably the most popular. They have been mentioned because they were at the forefront of the Christian healing revival of recent decades and because they illustrate one of its most important characteristics. While Kuhlman and Roberts both had strong ties to established churches in their backgrounds and neither ever provoked any conflict with them, their ministries were to a large extent independent. And while their ministries were wholeheartedly Christian, they picked up on one element in the Christian tradition, healing, which was being almost wholly ignored by mainstream Christian churches.

Mainstream Protestant and Catholic churches in the 1950s were very aware of the popularity of the healing revivalists, but reactions of clergy and theologians ranged from outright condemnation of the revivalists to condemnation of the churches themselves for neglecting the healing ministry. During the mid-1950s, the journal *Christian Century* and the National Council of Churches repeatedly attacked the healing revivalists, calling them racketeers and religious quacks.[41] Some theologians mounted sophisticated doctrinal arguments against faith healing, pointing out the redeeming qualities of suffering and "the lessons of adversity."[42] On the other hand, there were substantial numbers of clergy who recognized the popularity of the revivalists, Christian Science, and even spiritual healers as symptoms of neglect of the healing ministry by the church. The famous 1958 report of the Archbishop's Commission of the Church of England stated this explicitly:

The measure of the growth of these movements is to some extent the measure of the Church's failure to convince the world of important Christian truths. Where any part of the Catholic Faith has been minimized, where the whole gospel of Christ has not been preached, there sects have always flourished. Had the Church faithfully and intelligently carried out our Lord's commission to heal, Christian Science would have had no reason for existence.[43]

And as Father Francis MacNutt has written more recently:

These shrines and popular evangelistic services draw the same kind of crowds that Jesus attracted in his lifetime: wounded people who cry out along the roadside asking to be healed. . . . Admittedly, these devotions are often sentimental, sometimes superstitious, and frequently embarrassingly commercialized. But, I believe, this all came about because the prayers for material and physical needs were moved from the center of the life of the Church and were shunted aside into the area of popular devotion. It was as if theologians moved off in one direction, while the simple people with their basic needs moved off in another.[44]

This is a fairly common interpretation, then, that people who are sick will seek religious healing and, if this is unavailable to them in the church to which they belong, will go elsewhere for it.[45] The recent increasing receptiveness of the mainstream churches to healing ministries is an important historical change in the tradition of the Christian church.

One reason for the change may have to do with the increasing interest of the middle class in religious healing. It is true that the early followings of the healing revivalists were largely among the rural poor, who may well have had few other options in caring for their illnesses. The most successful of the revivalists, however, especially Roberts and Kuhlman, drew followers from the urban and suburban middle classes, who sought religious healing in addition to professional medical care. The impact of these revivalists was felt by all the major Protestant denominations.[46]

Another probable reason for the growth of interest in religious healing is the significant shift in morbidity patterns since the turn of the century. Chronic diseases, which make up the largest proportion of sickness in our society, are the very sorts of conditions for which people are likely to seek alternative treatments. Though this is not a subject religious writers have tended to comment on, the cases in a study of spiritual healing in Chicago area churches in 1954, and those mentioned in Kuhlman's famous book *I Believe in Miracles,* did tend to be largely healings of chronic illnesses.[47] Of course these cases prove nothing at all, except that such cures are more likely to be seen as miraculous. In fact, the little research available shows that it is a misconception to think that religious healing is sought only in the face of incurable disease or only after medical resources have been exhausted.[48] Nevertheless, it stands to reason that people will try more different remedies, including religious healing, for chronic conditions that are neither self-limiting nor easily controlled by medical treatment. And these are precisely the kinds of diseases that are on the increase.

A third possible source of the growth of interest in religious healing is concomitant with the second. The reason people seek more different remedies for chronic or non-self-limiting illness is that medical treatment, even when available and affordable, may not be completely satisfactory. For most chronic conditions, medical treatment is expensive because it is long term, and by definition it is not completely effective, in the sense of total cure, or the condition would not be chronic. Furthermore, medical effectiveness is reduced for chronic conditions by its failure to provide meaning for the experience of continued suffering. In fact, according to Kleinman, it is just this inability or unwillingness of modern medicine to provide meaning for the experience of illness that is causing what he calls "traditional healing activities" to surface in the wider social structure.[49] As medicine is increasingly viewed as impersonal, more humanistic or spiritual ways of dealing with illness are sought and may be used simultaneously with medical therapy.

It does make some historical sense, then, that interest in religious healing should be widespread at this time, when chronic conditions are becoming more prevalent. But it should be clear from the discussion of the place of healing in Jesus' ministry and subsequent Christian tradition that the phenomenon of mental and physical healing is very much a part of Christian tradition, not at all a perversion of it. Indeed, it is somewhat remarkable, given the undeniably central role of healing in the New Testament, that it has been neglected for so long. One suspects that a strong element in the enthusiasm and joy that accompany contemporary accounts of healing is the rediscovery of something new in what was old and familiar.

Any discussion of healing in American churches today, however, risks oversimplification if some important qualifications are not made. Though there has been an undeniable revival of interest in religious healing since the 1950s, the church had never abandoned its ministry to the sick, the troubled, and the dying. And while some churches may be far more willing than others to recognize or institute charismatic healing ministries, there are none that do not recognize the special claim of the sick to the care of the clergy and the congregation. Thus, although it would be impossible to predict the extent of healing activities in any given church, it is safe to say that all Christians regard some form of ministry to the sick as an essential part of their belief system. Nor can any easy generalizations be made about Catholic versus Protestant involvement with healing, since there are as many differences within these churches as there are between them. For the sake of clarity, however, we discuss the two separately. The remainder of this section is devoted to a brief description of healing activities and ministries to the sick commonly found in mainstream Protestant churches and some current theological perspectives on healing. The final section of this chapter is an in-depth look at a particular group of Roman Catholics for whom healing has taken on a vital new importance.

## Healing Activities in Mainstream Protestant Churches

Religious healing activities vary a great deal from one Protestant denomination to another. Since 1960 five of the major church bodies have published official studies of religious healing and the needs that exist for it today.[50] Undoubtedly the most common church ministry to the sick to be found in all denominations is visitation, by both clergy and congregation. The pastor or member of a congregation who visits the sick who are shut in at home or in the hospital demonstrates Christian concern, especially when a prayer is offered. Even if such prayers are offered in a general way, without any expectation of miraculous healing, they demonstrate quite graphically the sick person's membership in the Christian community, a community that transcends space and time. And as we have shown earlier, such social support can have real healing consequences.[51] It would be a mistake to assume that all, or even most, pastoral calls to the sick are made with any expectation that demonstrable healing will result. Our argument has been that, even where such expectations are lacking, the pastoral call reasserts the vitality of the mediating structure, which includes the social body of the church and the spiritual body of the wider Christian community. The wholeness of these bodies is communicated to the bodies of the sick.

A second widely dispersed healing resource of the Protestant churches is pastoral counseling, an age-old phenomenon that is increasingly viewed by both church and medical professionals as a community mental health resource. Community mental health studies have repeatedly shown that people at all income and educational levels used clergy counseling resources for help with life problems.[52] Gerald Gurin, Joseph Veroff, and Sheila Feld found that 42 percent of the people in their study of mental health sought help from a clergyman for a personal problem more often than from any other resource.[53] Such counseling has numerous and distinct advantages over professional mental health counseling, beginning with the fact that it is more widely available, both geographically and economically. For the most part clergy, unless they have had additional professional mental health training, do not charge fees, and going to see the pastor about a problem carries none of the stigma of mental illness. The potential for avoiding the iatrogenic effects of such labeling should be clear. Moreover, clergy have personal and spiritual relationships with troubled people and their families that enable them to share joys as well as sorrows. Clergy are also familiar with the ways their parishioners solve their problems. Furthermore, the pastor, unlike the mental health professional, does not have to wait for individuals to seek him or her out. He is expected to call on all members of the congregation.[54] Moreover, the religious quality of such counseling offers a special benefit to those seeking a spiritual dimension in their care.[55]

A third type of healing ministry found most commonly, but not exclusively, in the Episcopalian churches is the regular public healing service. These are frequently held at midweek, often in the middle of the day. Notices of such services frequently appear in the church announcement columns in the newspaper and are open to both members of the church and nonmembers. The service of prayers, hymns, and scripture reading may or may not include communion, but usually concludes with the laying on of hands for those who seek it. Such regularly held services, led by the priest or minister of the church, are usually quite unsensational.

The other type of healing service, which need not always be held in a church, is the healing revival mission. These services are led by healing evangelists whose reputations often draw large crowds, just as the tent revivalists of the 1950s did.

A final manifestation of the church's healing mission is the small prayer group, made up of concerned members of the church. Such a group may meet regularly to pray for the sick in the congregation, who may or may not be present. They may even pray for others at long distances or keep up a twenty-four-hour prayer vigil by taking turns.[56]

Of course not all Protestant churches have healing services or healing prayer groups, and some clergy are more willing than others to devote themselves to pastoral counseling. We have simply tried to show that Christian concern for the sick is expressed in several different activities of mainstream Protestant churches in our society today. We have also tried to suggest that the church is a mediator of healing even when it does not have an active healing ministry, though such ministries seem to be growing in numbers and importance. Even when a highly developed healing ministry has become centrally important to the life of a church, the church still exemplifies one of the primary qualities of a mediating structure: its multifunctionality. Church members who meet to pray for the sick experience a shared fellowship for themselves. Those who go to visit the shut-in may bring food along for the family, help care for a child whose parent is sick, or do other household chores. This multifunctionality, besides promoting the vitality of the social group, puts illness, healing, and caring into a larger context of spiritual beliefs and practical concerns.

### Protestant Theological Perspectives on Healing

We have said before that one essential aspect of healing is the provision of meaning for the experience of illness. All religions serve the purpose of establishing a religious interpretation of reality and locating important human experiences, including illness, within it. Christians have an extraordinarily rich tradition to draw on in interpreting suffering, illness, and death. As we saw earlier, Christian theological perspectives on illness have been anything but consistent over time or from one group to another. For some, religious healing has been the primary act of faith, whereas others have found strengthened faith through suffering, both views having a strong theological tradition behind them. Christianity speaks extensively to the problem of human suffering.

Contemporary Christian theological perspectives on healing have two strong elements in the tradition to draw on, two strands that strongly complement and reinforce each other. These may be called the power of God's love to heal and the redemptiveness of the act of suffering. Current theological debates on the place of healing in the church have pointed out the overemphasis on the tradition of redemption and the neglect of the healing power of Christian love.

The key to understanding the theological tradition of healing is in the life of Jesus Christ. Christians believe that Jesus was the son of God and the son of man as well. He was both fully divine and fully human, so that he shared all the experiences of human life. The early Christians believed in the essential good of the human body, soul, and life on this earth, and this was continually affirmed for them by Jesus' and the disciples' healing of the sick. Not only were the human body and soul both good, they were seen as inseparable, both worthy of love and healing. Jesus' ministry was to restore the whole of man, body and mind as well as soul. More than any other world religion, the Judeo-Christian tradition places value in this world, the physical body, and human relationships, giving it the potential to deal most fully with the problem of illness.[57]

Christian theologians who have written on the problem of sickness have generally agreed that sickness and suffering are evils to be overcome and that they do have some connection with sin. It is true that there is a close biblical association between healing and casting out evil spirits, indicating that, at least in the minds of the early Christians, there was identification of sickness with evil forces at work in the world.[58] Another manifestation of evil in human life is sin. Sickness can be and frequently is interpreted as the consequence of sin. Most theologians would argue against the notion that individual events of sickness could or should be seen as causally related to individual sinful acts. Rather, sin is usually defined more generally as a state of broken relations between God and man, a state of disorder that has existed since the Fall of Man.[59] And restoration of those right relations is therefore necessary if real healing, a return to wholeness, is to take place.

Some writers have seen in illness the opening up of new possibilities for salvation. Seeing illness as "a voice for the purpose of our healing"[60] is very different from seeing it as a cross that must be borne. Thus, they conclude, it should be normative for Christians to pray for the removal of sickness rather than accepting it for its redemptive value.[61] This argument, that sickness is the result of man's broken relationship with God, makes it incumbent on Christians to seek salvation by restoring the relationship. Thus the first thing that a liturgy of healing requires is confession, followed by repentance and forgiveness.

Ultimately, however, the Christian meaning of illness is inseparable from the Christian meaning of death, which many have called God's final healing.[62] The real meaning of Jesus' life is found not only in his healing of others but in his own overcoming of suffering and death so that all believers could have eternal life. Thus it was not a complete perversion of the Christian tradition that rites for healing were metamorphosed into last rites. The Christian meaning of healing does include easing the soul into eternal life. Christians can pray for healing for the dying and find their prayers answered.


## Sacraments of Healing

There are two aspects of Christian healing, which should be carefully distinguished from one another. Healing may be either sacramental or charismatic, though frequently these forms occur together. Charismatic healing is seen as a gift of the Holy Spirit and is commonly mediated through an individual who is believed to have a gift for healing. Sacramental healing, on the other hand, is mediated through a group receiving the sacraments, especially the Eucharist, the laying on of hands, and anointing with oil, and is far more common. The effect of prayer and the confession and forgiveness of sins is to create a meditative space around the illness and give it a full measure of religious meaning. The sacramental rites then bring the healer and the healed into a conscious and deliberate relation to God. The efficacy of the sacraments is by no means limited to those who are believed to have healing gifts.

Healing ministries in mainstream Protestant churches are most likely to be of the sacramental type, though they may be limited to prayer, confession, and the Eucharist. Laying on of hands and anointing with oil are practiced much less frequently. The Reformation largely abandoned the formal healing rituals of laying on of hands and anointing with oil, which are a strong part of the New Testament tradition. The importance of these sacraments lies in their ability to speak to the sick at a level deeper than consciousness.[63] The sacraments are not simply symbols; those that involve the physical body through touch bring the bodies of the sick into healing relationship with the rest of the community of Christians.

The laying on of hands occupied a crucially important place in the life of the early Christians but had fallen into almost complete disuse until the healing revival of the 1950s. It is now a regular part of church services in many Episcopalian churches, and it is being revived in other denominations, at times in untraditional forms, such as circles where hands are laid on all around. Some scientific experiments with the biological effects of the laying on of hands have been done with mice, in which it appeared that the wounds of mice treated with laying on of hands healed more quickly than wounds that were not so treated.[64] Of course, the symbolic significance of the act was probably lost on the mice, so there are apparently some physiological effects as well. This very human gesture manages to combine the simple physical warmth of touch with an emotional warmth of caring and concern. It symbolizes sympathy and contact, and it focuses the immediate experience of healer and healed in a very real way. Physical touch also conveys to the sick an openness and acceptance of their condition, which they may perceive as their own uncleanness or imperfection.[65]

The Eucharist, or Holy Communion, is the central sacrament of the Christian church and carries heavy symbolic and emotional significance. The early Christians found spontaneous healings occurring during celebrations of the Eucharist, even when the sick were not singled out for laying on of hands or Holy Unction.[66] The Church of England today recommends that Holy Communion be celebrated whenever a healing service is conducted in the church, so as to connect it closely with the healing ministry. Holy Communion is the act of Christians, members of the church, sharing with each other and taking into themselves symbols of the body of Christ. Perhaps even more than the laying on of hands, the sharing of Holy Communion has the potential for transmitting to the body of the believer the strength, vitality, and connectedness of the larger body of the church.

Anointing with oil, or Holy Unction, was also a practice of the early Christians. Though there is no scriptural record of Jesus anointing the sick, it is probable that he did and certain that his disciples did. It was at the time a widely accepted therapeutic technique that acquired Christian significance through the accompanying prayers. There were several traditional approaches to anointing. The simplest was to anoint the head or breast as the seat of the soul, from which the healing effects could radiate. Alternatively, each extremity was anointed so that the effects could converge at the center. Another method was to anoint the place of greatest weakness or ailment. At times simply the hands were anointed. Finally, the dominant practice became the anointing the five senses to purify them.[67] Recently the Roman Catholic Church, in its 1974 pronouncement "Anointing of the Sick," changed its practice, from anointing the five senses for forgiveness of their sins, to anointing the head and hands. This is just one of a number of changes in the anointing of the sick that have transformed it from primarily a rite of forgiveness for the dying to a sacrament for healing in this life.[68]

The other type of healing, charismatic healing, may also involve the administration of sacraments, particularly the laying on of hands. The Eucharist may be administered only by ordained clergy, who may or may not have charismatic healing gifts. Anointing with oil is also limited by some denominations to administration by those who are ordained. The charismatic healer, however, possesses a gift for healing that is independent of the sacraments. This charism, or gift of the Holy Spirit, is an endowment recognized since the early church and acknowledged by both Roman Catholics and Protestants. Charismatic healing among contemporary Roman Catholics will be looked at later, but there is also a strong tradition of Protestant charismatic healers, including Kathryn Kuhlman,[69] Oral Roberts, William Branham,[70] Agnes Sanford,[71] Ruth Carter Stapleton,[72] and Emily Gardiner Neal.[73] Such people are recognized as peculiarly receptive channels for God's healing power. Those who have written about their gifts have taken pains to deny that there is anything special about them as individuals that gives them the ability to heal, and they frequently assure readers that any believer could do what they do. This is somewhat paradoxical, given the extraordinary nature of some of the healings recounted in these books. These accounts of healing often mention actual sensations experienced by both the healer and the healed that are described as being like a surge of warmth or a flow of electricity channeled through the laying on of hands to the head or the most afflicted part of the body.

But the most important thing about Christian healing, whether it is charismatic and miraculous or sacramental and simply comforting, is that it speaks to the human condition at all its levels. The combination of physical touch, eating and drinking, and anointing with oil with the self-reflection of the confession of sins and the prayers and praise of God makes for a very powerful interpretation of the experience of illness. Christian healing speaks to all levels of human consciousness, physical, emotional (both conscious and unconscious), and spiritual. Given the complexity of the theology involved and the infinite range of life situations in which people find themselves when they are ill, the potential clearly exists for people to find individually meaningful and satisfying interpretations for the difficult reality of illness. More important, those interpretations are made in the context of a religious community surrounding the sick person that has both an earthly immediacy and an immortal reality.

## A CLOSER LOOK: HEALING IN THE CATHOLIC CHARISMATIC RENEWAL

The Catholic Charismatic Renewal movement began in this country in 1967. It has since become a full-fledged international movement within the Roman Catholic Church. Though it is not originally or primarily a healing movement, healing is recognized as one among the many gifts of the Holy Spirit that Catholic Charismatics are given to exercise. We have chosen to look at it in detail here for a number of reasons. First, the movement is widespread and obviously significant in the lives of large numbers of people. Second, there is some good literature and research available on the activity of healing, originating both within the movement and in more objective, social scientific sources.

Religious healing among Catholic Charismatics, or Pentecostals, is a familiar activity. It is part of their religious reality. Although it is recognized as a significant sign of God's love and hence a cause for joy, even excitement, it is not treated at all sensationally or as a rare curiosity. Accounts of healings, even of serious illnesses, have become relatively common in Catholic Charismatic publications and at meetings, and as they become more common they become more expected. As we shall see, Catholic Charismatic healing is based on a set of religiously informed beliefs and practices about health and illness that, while they may not be shared with other religious groups or the culture as a whole, are consistent and are shared by a large number of American Roman Catholics. This is a significant new nonprofessional source of health care.

The Catholic Charismatic Renewal, or Catholic Pentecostalism (the names are interchangeable), began among a group of people at Duquesne University in Pittsburgh, Pennsylvania, in 1967. Students and faculty of the Roman Catholic university were attending a weekend retreat in February when a number of them began to pray for and received "baptism in the Holy Spirit."[74] The thirty people who had been present spread the news quickly, and three weeks later more baptisms in the Spirit occurred at a weekend retreat at the University of Notre Dame. Other, similar outpourings began to occur across the country. In April 1967 more than eighty people traveled to Notre Dame for a weekend retreat that spread the experience even further. There have been annual meetings or conferences at Notre Dame every year since then, and the attendance has grown, from 100 in 1968, to 4,500 in 1971, to 30,000 in 1974.[75]

Healing, which had always been regarded by Protestant Pentecostals as one of the gifts of the Holy Spirit, was, interestingly, not emphasized at all by the early leaders of the Catholic Charismatic movement.[76] One writer commented in 1971 that Catholic prayer groups were not as "preoccupied" as Protestant Pentecostal groups with the subject of healing.[77] The healings that occurred were welcomed as signs of God's love, but they tended not to be sought directly. A noticeable change in the attitudes of the leaders of the movement toward the healing ministry first became obvious at the 1974 Notre Dame Conference.[78] On the first day of that conference, about 30,000 people attended a healing service led by three of the now-recognized leaders of the healing ministry of the Catholic Charismatic Renewal—Father Francis MacNutt, Father Mike Scanlan, and Barbara Shlemon. About seventy physical healings were reported immediately, including cases of blindness, arthritis, cancer, back problems, deafness, blood disease, and others. The movement's magazine, *New Covenant,* has since printed numerous testimonies of healings that occurred at the conference, including cases of coronary heart disease, narcolepsy, rheumatoid arthritis, and epilepsy.[79] Since that time the healing ministry has acquired increasing importance in the movement, judging from the spate of articles on healing that began to appear in *New Covenant* and the number of books that began to be published.[80]

The basic unit of the Catholic Charismatic Renewal is, however, not the mass rally, but the local prayer group, and this is where most healing activities take place. The prayer group meets regularly and may be made up of from 3 to 1,000 members, the median number being 28.[81] The *International Directory of Catholic Charismatic Prayer Groups,* which listed slightly more than 1,000 such groups in the United States in 1973, listed more than 4,500 in the United States and Canada in 1980.[82] Such groups first began to be formed on college campuses, among graduate students and faculty, especially in Indiana and Michigan. A substantial proportion of the movement continues to be centered in university communities, although the movement has spread well beyond the university. Nationally recognized leaders of the movement are nearly all university trained and associated, and the general level of education of the members of prayer groups still tends to be quite high.

One study of prayer groups in the Ann Arbor, Michigan area revealed their rather solidly middle-class membership.[83] Catholic students at the University of Michigan who had joined Pentecostal prayer groups did not differ in socioeconomic background from Catholic students who did not join. Nearly half the nonstudent members were college graduates, and well over half had white-collar jobs or spouses with white-collar jobs. Another study of non-university-centered prayer groups in northern New Jersey revealed the same high level of involvement by the middle class.[84] Sixty percent of the nonstudent members were housewives, 20 percent white-collar workers, and 20 percent blue-collar workers. The average age of nonstudents in these groups was fifty-five, and women outnumbered men by two to one. The vast majority of participants in the prayer groups in both studies were active, practicing Catholics before their involvement with the prayer groups, and both studies showed high participation by priests and nuns, who were often the effective leaders of the groups. Thus, although no national data are available on the socioeconomic characteristics of people who join prayer groups, available data suggest that the membership, student and nonstudent, is drawn largely from the well-educated middle class. The international directory does include the percentage of each prayer group's membership that is Catholic, which is almost uniformly 80 to 100 percent. The authors of both studies conclude that the Catholic Pentecostal movement arose not in response to economic deprivation or political disenfranchisement, but in reaction to tensions felt within the Catholic Church and on college campuses during the 1960s.[85] McGuire specifically relates the movement to feelings of malaise among Catholics who feel the order and authority of the Catholic Church shaken in the wake of Vatican II. The Pentecostal movement, according to this interpretation, satisfies a need for security and authority beyond those made available by human social institutions, which are evidently subject to change. That timeless security and authority are being found in the direct experience of the Holy Spirit, whether it be through baptism in the Holy Spirit, speaking in tongues, or healing.

As mentioned earlier, the early leaders of the movement did not regard healing as one of the most important gifts of the Holy Spirit. At most it was an incidental side effect of being filled with the Holy Spirit, something to praise God for but not something to be actively sought. At the least there was some open skepticism and hesitation about praying for healing, an activity still closely associated with the perceived anti-intellectual emotionalism of the Protestant Pentecostal "faith healers" of the 1950s.[86] But these attitudes have changed considerably since 1974, and prayers for healing are now a regular part of most prayer group meetings.

Catholic Pentecostals recognize that gifts of healing are not evenly distributed among individuals, even among those who have received baptism in the Holy Spirit. Just as some people sing better than others, so some have a special gift for healing. Nevertheless, all Catholic Pentecostals are exhorted to pray for their friends and relatives who are sick.[87]

Prayers for healing of the sick take place in many contexts: privately, at special visits to the sick at home or in the hospital, at home-centered "share" groups, at regular meetings of the prayer group, at special healing masses, and at mass rallies. Laurentin makes an important distinction between the objective and subjective aspects of the spiritual experience of Pentecostals at these meetings, which especially applies to the experience of healing. He distinguishes the interior transformation called "baptism in the Spirit" from the external exercise of the gifts of the Spirit in the service of others.[88] The experiences of healing and being healed differ in the same way. But both bring the participants a new sense of the presence of God, restoring the healer's and the healed person's relationships to God. The ultimate goal of the healing service, then, is not the healing of individual physical or emotional ills, but the worship of God by the community of Christians. Laurentin calls the exercise of the gifts of the Holy Spirit an attempt to recapture the enthusiasm and inspiration of the early Church.[89] It is certainly an attempt to bring direct religious experience back into the lives of middle-class Catholics.

Before looking at the healing practices of these groups, it would be helpful to have an idea of the place of health and illness in the Catholic Pentecostal world view. Though only one research project has been undertaken in an attempt to outline these ideas as they are held by ordinary members of prayer groups,[90] there is substantial agreement between these views, revealed in interviews, letters, testimonies, and articles published in *New Covenant,* and the more scholarly writings of the movement's leaders. Thus it is possible to outline a set of beliefs about health and illness that, though not formalized in any doctrinal sense, form a shared backdrop of meanings for the activities of healing.

Any group's notion of health tends to embody its ideals for individual and social life. And notions of illness represent failures to approximate that ideal. Not surprisingly, Catholic Pentecostals who have been questioned about their definitions of health nearly all included spiritual criteria in their definition, and that tended to be framed in terms of the individual's relationship with God.[91] In the groups studied, the most frequently mentioned criterion of health was "oneness with the Lord." In fact, spiritual criteria for health superseded physical criteria in importance, many respondents asserting that it was perfectly possible to be physically unwell and still truly healthy. In fact, when asked, only one member of the prayer groups mentioned any criterion for health that was at all physical (being full of energy), and even that was heavily psychological. Other criteria mentioned were spiritual, moral, emotional, psychological, or social. Though it should not be surprising that a religious group, especially one with an interest in healing, would have a basically religious definition of what health is, it should cause one to pause and reflect how radically different these criteria are from medical or even psychological norms. According to this definition, for example, it is not possible for an atheist to be healthy.

Illness, then, for Catholic Pentecostals, is any state of physical or emotional brokenness that includes a broken relationship with God. The origins of illness in the Catholic Pentecostal world view are complex, however, reflecting the complexity of the theology involved. The question of the causes of illness is one that occupies most people who experience serious illness, but it is particularly difficult for people who are, or think of themselves as, "good Christians." That is, it is difficult for faithful Christians to reconcile their continued suffering with their belief in a God of power and love. MacNutt has devoted considerable space in his two books to answering these questions, and his writings can be considered somewhat authoritative. According to him, the source of all sickness is sin, understood as a broken relationship with God, which has been the state of the human condition since the Fall. To be more specific, there are three levels at which sickness may afflict people. Sickness of the spirit is caused directly by personal sin; emotional sickness is caused by emotional hurts from an individual's personal relationships; and physical sickness is caused by disease or accidents. In addition, any of these three basic types of sickness can be caused by demonic forces.[92]

MacNutt has developed an elaborate theodicy, or explanation for the existence of evil in the world, which he sees so plainly manifested as sickness. He finds that original sin is not an abstraction but a real affliction that people should not be blamed for. He counsels the sick and their families by emphasizing that sickness is the work of an enemy and that it is an evil to be overcome, not to be righteously suffered. Sickness and suffering elude human understanding; they are part of the mystery of evil; so they can be overcome only by an intelligence and power that go beyond what any human beings possess. Thus praying for healing is not merely one choice Christians may exercise. It is actually incumbent on them to seek God's help in times of sickness.[93]

McGuire's study of the beliefs about health and illness held by the members of prayer groups shows that they hold a remarkably similar, if less theologically sophisticated, point of view. She points out that constructing an explanation for an event of illness is an intrinsic part of the process of healing and that such explanations organize physical and social events in meaningful ways that allow the illness to make sense to the sufferer and his family. Because Catholic Pentecostals have such elaborate beliefs about health and illness, the interpretation of the causes of an individual's illness serves the purpose of linking him with the larger meaning system of this entire social group.[94]

McGuire's respondents were questioned about general causes of illness and the causes of specific illnesses they had themselves experienced. In her interviews, the most frequently cited cause of disease, mentioned by more than two-thirds of those questioned, was "sin," meaning both a general condition of being "out of order" and a reference to personal, sinful acts. For many of the respondents, definitions of illness and causes of illness were indistinguishable; in other words, "that which they need to be healed of is perceived to be part of the cause of illness." It was the sin itself that brought on the illness directly, not God who punished sinful acts with sickness. Yet they did recognize several levels of responsibility with regard to sin, personal sin implying much greater responsibility for the resulting illness than the general state of being "out of order" with God.[95]

The second most common cause of illness was evil spirits, mentioned as important by one-fourth of the respondents. Here, too, there was some distinction made as to the extent of individual responsibility: for some, these evil forces were completely beyond human control; for others, they gained power over an individual through a weakness in his emotional or spiritual life.[96]

A third category encompassed the effects of the social, physical, and emotional environment on the individual and implied only moderate responsibility. Examples of these sorts of conditions are environmental pollutants, poverty, war, difficult childhood experiences, and job stress. Finally, there was the category for accidents, for which the individual was seen as having very little responsibility. These conditions included birth defects and physical accidents.[97]

Certainly for these respondents any event of illness could have more than one cause, just as the illnesses themselves could have emotional, physical and spiritual dimensions. MacNutt, too, discusses illness in terms of multiple causation, though with considerable conceptual clarity. This type of "diagnosis" is necessary not just for the benefit of personal interpretation, for then these categories would be purely formal. The main function of determining the cause of an illness is to determine the type of healing necessary.

By and large, the practice of healing among Catholic Pentecostals is highly traditional, in a scriptural sense and in terms of the traditions of the Catholic Church. The one significant innovation that has been made by Pentecostal Catholics, which distinguishes them even from the earlier Protestant healing revivalists, is the recognition of four types of healing, which correspond to MacNutt's four categories of illness causation. Although it was MacNutt who first wrote about it, the typology appears to have emerged from the movement spontaneously as people specialized in one variety of healing or another.

Healing for physical illness is, according to MacNutt, "the simplest kind of prayer." He advises first listening to those in need in order to know what to pray for. Knowing when and what to pray for is itself a gift of the Holy Spirit, often called discernment. It involves both the interpretation of the sufferer, prompted or directed by those who are going to pray, and their own perception of God's will in the matter. This gift may come as simple intuition, or it may even take a physical form, such as the sensation of warmth or a mild flow of "electricity." Knowing what to pray for is easier for healing a physical illness with obvious symptoms, but MacNutt warns healing ministers that more than one type of healing may be necessary and listening is very important. The prayer for healing that follows usually, but not necessarily, is said with the laying on of hands. The sensation that accompanies discernment often accompanies the laying on of hands, making it feel to both parties as if a "gentle electric current" were flowing. There is some biblical support for the interpretation that Jesus experienced just such a flow of power, as in the case of the woman who was bleeding.[98]

Not everyone experiences this physical sensation, however, and healings are said to take place without the occurrence of any sensations. The actual prayer usually includes an invoking of the presence of God, a petition for healing, and then closes with a thanksgiving. Prayers are usually short, simple, and direct, including the person's name but not necessarily any specific information about the illness.[99]

The second type of healing, for emotional or mental problems, is commonly called "inner healing" or "healing of the memories." There are a large number of books and articles devoted to this type of healing, and all usually involve emotional problems stemming from past hurts that have never been successfully resolved. The healing of these past hurts is accomplished by, first, a talking through of the problem, going back through the person's biography and discussing key events related to the present trouble. This is followed by prayer to heal the hurtful effects of those events, which may be manifesting themselves as compulsion, neurosis, anxiety, or depression.[100] Some writers have seen inner healing as occurring more easily and often than physical healing.[101] Others have outlined complex processes through which the sufferers relive their experiences and forgive those who had hurt them.[102] The parallel to secular psychotherapy is obvious, and indeed some of the same processes are probably at work in both cases, but their differences are also significant;[103] inner healing should be seen as different even from conventional religiously oriented psychotherapy.[104]

The third type of healing is the one MacNutt considers most important. Spiritual sickness is a broken relationship with God resulting from sinful acts. Spiritual sickness can and often does have physical manifestations. Though MacNutt cautions against playing amateur psychologist and imputing sinfulness to all those who are sick, he does advise, on the basis of scripture, that repentance and prayers for forgiveness are often appropriate in accompanying prayers for physical healing. According to MacNutt, the most important form of repentance is the forgiveness of others "who trespass against us." There is some sort of bargain at work here; those who cannot forgive wrongs done to them cannot have their own sins forgiven. Bitterness, resentment, or anger toward others are sins in themselves, though they may begin as responses to others' sins. Thus the first condition for being forgiven is to forgive others. For a spiritual sickness, only a spiritual healing can be effective.[105]

The final type of healing is quite different from the others, and MacNutt is one of the few who discuss it at all. He distinguishes demonic *possession,* which requires formal exorcism, from demonic *oppression,* which is far more common and requires only prayer for deliverance. Either of these two states can produce disturbing behavior patterns and mental states that may be diagnosed as schizophrenia or psychosis. (He does *not* argue that all mental illness is demonic.) There is considerable biblical support for the practice in the healings of Jesus and his disciples.[106] Unlike prayers for healing, prayers for deliverance are directed at the demons rather than at God and take the form of a command rather than a petition. They are also said "in the name of Jesus Christ" and are thus invested with his authority. MacNutt cautions that only those experienced in this type of ministry should undertake it, and then only with a team, since unusual occurrences apparently still occur. Hence the prayer for deliverance usually also includes a plea for protection for those present.[107]

One further word on these four types of healing strategies. Catholic Pentecostal healing contains elements of all these types of healing, which may not be at all clearly distinguished from one another in practice. Indeed, given the emphasis on wholeness and oneness with God, it would be surprising if physical conditions were seen as wholly separate from emotional or spiritual health. Thus it might seem as if these classifications, both of the types of illnesses and of their corresponding healings, were simply academic. They are not. The classification is an "emic" one, that is, one that was received or developed and is used by the members of a social group to interpret their experiences.[108] Except, perhaps, for some of the techniques of inner healing, there are strong scriptural parallels for all the activities involved in the different types of healing. Furthermore, the written classifications originated with those most heavily involved in the healing ministry. And these people not only practice healing, they teach others to pray for healing and write books and magazine articles that are widely read by Catholic Pentecostals.

The actual elements of the healing ministry among Catholic Pentecostals are not much different from those used in Protestant churches. The ministry involves both gifts (charisms) and sacraments, though of course there is more emphasis on the charisms. The healing ministry is never practiced in isolation but always in the context of a community, most usually the local prayer group or at least the local prayer group leaders. In McGuire's study of healing ministries among prayer groups in New Jersey, she found that those groups with the most highly developed prayer ministries often had special prayer rooms where the ministry team would meet with people to pray for all sorts of problems, especially for healings. These meetings usually consisted of a statement of the problem by the person seeking help, then prayers of praise and petition as to how to deal with the problem. Sometimes counseling takes place, or scripture reading, or further discussion. The prayer for healing may be quite specific, if some discernment of what to pray for has been received. Otherwise it may be a quite general prayer, or it may be spoken in tongues. Hands are laid on the head, arms, shoulders, or the affected part of the body. These meetings and prayers may be repeated as often as they are felt to be necessary.[109]

The gift of discernment is a very powerful gift not given to all those who pray for the sick, but it does enable those who receive it to know the cause of the illness and hence when to pray, what to pray for, and when to stop. The gift of discernment allows the receiver to know what God's will is in a particular situation. It may even take on the extreme form of knowledge that it is God's will that a person die and that his physical healing is not to be prayed for.[110]

The prayer that does take place is an intercessory prayer; that is, it is prayed to God by someone of behalf of someone else. The "minister" of healing is then a mediator between the healing power of God and the supplicant, the individual who seeks healing.[111] The prayers may be very short or very long; they may sometimes go on for hours. MacNutt devotes considerable attention to the concept of "soaking prayer," which can mean either very long prayers or frequently repeated ones.[112] The name connotes a seeping through to the core of something that had been dry and needs to be revived. Such prayers are usually prayed for people who are seriously ill and need healing in many parts of their body or for people who have suffered from chronic illness for a long time. MacNutt advises ministers of healing to keep praying if signs of healing begin to appear, if pains lessen, or if functions begin to return. The prayer, if continued at one sitting, can be interspersed with silence, singing, or praying in tongues, all accompanied by constant laying on of hands. MacNutt makes some interesting observations about this kind of prayer, which requires a great investment of time by those doing the praying. This is the sort of prayer most likely to be offered by people who are in continuous relationship with each other. It obviously cannot be prayed by ministers of healing at public services. The most frequently given examples of soaking prayer, in fact, involve family members who pray for each other for weeks, months, even years. MacNutt advises families to learn to pray for the chronically ill in their families.[113]

The laying on of hands is the physical accompaniment of the

spiritual act of prayer for healing. Laurentin observes that all kinds of prayer in the Charismatic Renewal, not just those for healing, may have physical aspects. Charismatic Catholics may pray with their hands open and lifted up or prostrate face down on the ground or kneeling and bowing. These postures make the body an integral part of prayer, a practice more common in Eastern religions but one that has obvious relevance in prayer for healing.[114] The laying on of hands is not limited to prayer for healing. It is also helpful in obtaining the initial experience of "baptism in the Spirit," which is how it was first used by Catholic Pentecostals. But in addition to the elements of tradition, the importance of the laying on of hands lies in the *connection* that is made. It is a practical, sensible, concrete expression of solidarity that communicates concern and love in a language of its own.

Praying in tongues also frequently, but not necessarily, accompanies prayers for healing. This gift was manifested early in the Catholic Pentecostal movement, and though it remains somewhat controversial,[115] it also rests on a strong scriptural and historical basis. It is not treated at all sensationally, however, and MacNutt suggests that it be a part of the practice of "soaking prayer."[116]

These practices—discernment, prayer for four types of healing, laying on of hands, and praying in tongues—do distinguish Charismatic Catholics from other Roman Catholics. But Charismatic Catholics also find healing efficacy in the holy sacraments of the church, which are shared by all Roman Catholics. Three sacraments in particular—Anointing of the Sick, Penance, and the Eucharist—are directly intended for healing, and the Holy Orders enjoin priests to heal the sick. As mentioned before, Anointing the Sick, which used to be called Extreme Unction, or Last Rites, has recently been changed to emphasize healing rather than absolution. It is no longer reserved for those who are dying but is to be administered to all the seriously ill.[117] The sacrament of Penance also has recently undergone some changes that make it facilitate healing. Rather than confession of sins, new emphasis is being placed on the reconciliation of relationships. This sacrament is frequently administered with prayers for inner healing.[118] The Eucharist, too, has been given new healing emphasis by the Charismatic Renewal, though its association with healing goes back as far as the New Testament and the writings of St. Teresa of Avila.[119]

Catholic Charismatics have by no means rejected the sacramental forms of the Roman Catholic Church in favor of the free exercise of the gifts of the Spirit. These people were nearly all actively practicing Catholics before their involvement in the Renewal, and the majority have retained their close ties with their church.[120] Thus, while some of the forms of healing practices would be new to lifelong Catholics, others are just new emphases in traditional sacramental forms (some of which had been healing rites in the past) that give them a whole new meaning.

It should be clear by now that beliefs about health, illness, and healing occupy a position of considerable importance in the Catholic Pentecostal world view. Health and illness are so heavily invested with symbolic meaning that criteria for evaluating them are actually more spiritual than physical. It has been our argument throughout this book that personal interpretations of the meaning of illness are directly relevant to the means of healing sought. To go one step further, these interpretations are also relevant to the outcomes of healing strategies. In other words, if an individual believes the root cause of his illness to be a broken relationship with his parents, any healing strategy that treats him in isolation and concentrates on his physical symptoms will not meet his own criterion for healing. As we have seen, explanations for the causes of illness for Catholic Pentecostals stem primarily from unsatisfactory spiritual or social relationships; so it makes sense that healings would take place on those levels. The efficacy of religious healing, then, rests on its relevance to the individual's perception of the problem. Furthermore, this is a real, not just a definitional, efficacy. In spiritual healing, where sin is seen to be the direct cause of illness, the means actually exist for removing the cause, through penance and forgiveness. One really can be assured that one's sins will be forgiven. To the Pentecostal Catholic, healing means wholeness: "Health is holiness."[121]

All of this makes the question of medical verification of religious healing a thorny problem. Medical verification of miraculous religious healing does exist, as at Lourdes, for example, where the medical and spiritual criteria for healing miracles are so strict that very few cases actually qualify as miracles. Yet when, at public healing services, people are asked to indicate whether or not they have been healed, only 25 percent say that they have not been helped. Approximately 25 percent customarily say they have been completely healed, and 50 percent feel themselves to be improved.[122] The fact that there are all these people claiming to be healed can only be understood in the context of what illness and healing mean in the Catholic Pentecostal world view. Clearly there are different sets of criteria for healing, and few cases succeed equally by both medical and religious criteria. Thus there are conceptual problems of which social scientists studying these phenomena must be fully aware; chief among these is the tendency for social science to accept the medical construction of the reality of illness and healing as primary or somehow more real than the religious version. Certainly for Catholic Pentecostals the religious construction of this reality is primary, and any healings that are experienced within this definitional context only make it more real. Thus, to a certain extent, these claims of healings must be accepted on their own terms—the non–Catholic Pentecostal must realize that the criteria used for judging healing are quite different from medical criteria. For Catholic Pentecostals themselves, medical verification of healing is something of a side issue; it is not necessary to prove something "scientifically" to someone who already believes in it.

On the other hand, there is little or no antagonism between leaders of the Catholic Pentecostal healing ministry and the medical profession. Leaders of the healing ministry do not try to discredit medical treatment or undermine the relationship the sick person may have with a doctor. Again and again one reads in the literature that the sick should use all the means at their disposal to get well. Furthermore, those who have experienced healing following prayer are encouraged to return to their doctor to verify the healing and not to discontinue medication or treatment until the doctor permits it.[123] In other words, among Catholic Pentecostals there is a recognition of the legitimacy of the medical evaluation of health and the usefulness of medical treatment.

There is some minor criticism of medicine from healing ministers concerned with iatrogenesis; MacNutt commonly prays for people to be spared the side effects of medical treatment, especially chemotherapy and radiation treatment, but he softens it by likening such prayers to the Church practice of blessing the oil for anointing.[124] He does note, however, that prayers have no danger of producing harmful side effects and so can be as long and as frequent as desired.

For the Catholic Pentecostal, then, though the medical construction of reality may not be wrong, it is certainly not enough. A real healing must involve the sick person's relationships with his family and friends and with God. So religious healing is generally sought *in addition to*, not *instead of,* medical care. Catholic Pentecostals come mainly from the middle and working classes, as we have seen, groups for whom medical treatment is generally available and affordable. In addition, they have more than average education, another factor frequently associated with higher use of medical care. There is no reason to conclude that the use of prayers for healing is a choice made out of ignorance, fear, or lack of alternatives.

It seems clear that there is some deeply felt need being satisfied here, where religious reality comes to bear on the physical or mental reality of illness. The experience of the healing of a physical or emotional hurt in the context of a religious ritual must be acknowledged to be a powerful experience. In fact, the entire Catholic Pentecostal movement is founded on a search for direct religious experience through baptism in the Holy Spirit. The exercise of each of the charisms constitutes a religious experience, and these are actively sought by Catholic Pentecostals.[125] The effect of the exercise of any of the charisms is a strong confirmation of the power and nearness of God. And the faith of people who have spoken in tongues or felt surges of warmth or electricity flowing through their body is understandably strengthened. Even people who have not experienced the charisms themselves but have simply heard others speak in tongues or seen others "resting in the Spirit" are likely to call their experience a religious one. A healing, however, is not simply a positive religious experience, though an immediate physical sensation may indeed occur. A complete or even partial healing removes a pain or a grief that may have been of the most serious kind, causing the individual to reinterpret his whole life in the context of that single experience. Even a healing of a minor ailment acts to confirm belief. These are the kind of experiences that make people deeply religious. They constitute evidence for the reality of God against which few doubts can compete. The physical or emotional fact of a healing lives on after the experience of healing is over, making itself a powerful reminder. And apparently the number of Catholic Pentecostals experiencing healings continues to grow.

The relevance of these healing practices to a discussion of mediating structures does not rest on questions of individual faith, however, as important as they may be from the perspective of religion. More important is the fact that these activities take place in small, ongoing groups that meet regularly and often, whose members know each other and share a strong set of values. They may also share some very powerful experiences. Both studies of prayer groups mentioned found that the members of the groups valued very highly the community they had found.[126] The data from one study also suggested that the movement is more attractive to people who are lonely and seeking a religious community.[127] The Charismatic Catholic who belongs to such a community makes it a very important part of her life: the average respondent in one study spent five hours each week with Charismatics other than her family.[128]

These communities of Catholic Charismatics are a new phenomenon, just over thirteen years old. The practice of praying for healing within these groups is even more recent. But both seem to be affecting increasing numbers of people in all age groups.

There are a number of similarities between this movement and the home childbirth movement. Both charismatic healing and having babies at home are ancient practices that fell out of favor and are undergoing revivals. Both seem to be growing mainly, though not solely, among members of the middle class, who have a reasonably wide range of choices for professional medical care. These non-professional alternatives, then, are being chosen, not out of a lack of alternatives, but because they have something more to offer. Finally, both constitute a demand for a certain type of experience, one that is profound and binds very tightly together those who share in it. These experiences are deeply moving spiritually and emotionally, and strongly physical as well. They concern matters of utmost human importance—life and birth and death. The fact that people are deliberately creating the conditions for these experiences, and sharing them with those to whom they are closest indicates a desire to bring physical intimacy back into relationships whose basis is emotional or spiritual. This added dimension is surely a sign of the vitality of these groups and a source of their future strength.

## REFERENCES

1.  Peter Berger and Richard Neuhaus, *To Empower People* (Washington, D.C.: American Enterprise Institute, 1977), p. 27.
2.  Constant H. Jacquet, Jr., ed., *Yearbook of American and Canadian*

*Churches 1977* (Nashville: Abingdon Press, 1977), p. 244. The use of the term "church" in this chapter includes religious organizations of all faiths.

3. Gallup Opinion Index Report No. 145 (Princeton, N.J.: American Institute of Public Opinion, 1977–78), p. 22f.

4. Sydney E. Ahlstrom, *A Religious History of the American People* (New Haven, Conn.: Yale University Press, 1972), p. 952.

5. Gallup Opinion Index Report No. 145, p. 17.

6. Donald A. Tubesing, *An Idea in Evolution: History of the Wholistic Health Centers Project 1970-1976* (Hinsdale, Ill.: Wholistic Health Centers, 1976).

7. Michael J. Dowling, *Health Care and the Church* (Philadelphia: United Church Press, 1977).

8. Peter L. Berger, *The Sacred Canopy: Elements of a Sociological Theory of Religion* (Garden City, N.Y.: Doubleday, 1967), p. 25.

9. C.G. Jung, *Modern Man in Search of a Soul* (New York: Harcourt, Brace, 1933), p. 264.

10. See, for example, the Church of England Archbishop's Commission on Divine Healing, *The Church's Ministry of Healing* (Westminster: Church Information Board, 1958), pp. 11–12.

11. Arthur Kleinman, Leon Eisenberg, and Byron Good, "Culture, Illness, and Care: Clinical Lessons from Anthropological and Cross-Cultural Research," *Annals of Internal Medicine,* vol. 88 (1978), pp. 251-58.

12. Allan Young, "Some Implications of Medical Beliefs and Practices for Social Anthropology," *American Anthropologist* 78 (1976): 5-24.

13. Arthur M. Kleinman, "Some Issues for a Comparative Study of Medical Healing," *International Journal of Social Psychiatry,* 19 (1973): 159-65.

14. Jerome Frank, *Persuasion and Healing: A Comparative Study of Psychotherapy* (Baltimore: Johns Hopkins University Press, 1961), pp. 20-35.

15. Anthony Colson, "The Differential Use of Medical Resources in Developing Countries," *Journal of Health and Social Behavior* 12 (1971): 226-37.

16. Kleinman, Eisenberg and Good, "Culture, Illness, and Care," p. 252.

17. Meredith McGuire, *The Control of Charisma: A Sociological Interpretation of the Catholic Pentecostal Movement* (forthcoming).

18. Cyril C. Richardson, "Spiritual Healing in the Light of History," in Simon Doniger, ed., *Healing: Human and Divine* (New York: Association Press, 1957), pp. 206-16; A.H. Purcell Fox, *The Church's Ministry of Healing* (London: Longmans, Green, 1959), p. 47.

19. Kevin and Dorothy Ranaghan, *Catholic Pentecostals* (New York: Paulist Press, 1969), p. 204.

20. David Bakan, *Disease, Pain, and Sacrifice* (Boston: Beacon Press, 1968), p. vii.

21.  Max Weber, *The Sociology of Religion*, trans. Ephraim Fischoff (Boston: Beacon Press, 1964), chap. 9.

22.  Morton Kelsey, *Healing and Christianity: In Ancient Thought and Modern Times* (New York: Harper & Row, 1973), pp. 33–45.

23.  Ernest Becker, *The Denial of Death* (New York: Free Press, 1973), p. 90.

24.  Kelsey, *Healing and Christianity,* pp. 33–41. This is by far the best recent and widely available book on healing in Christian history and tradition.

25.  C.A. Meier, *Ancient Incubation and Modern Psychotherapy* (Evanston, Ill.: Northwestern University Press, 1967).

26.  Seward Hiltner, *Religion and Health* (New York: Macmillan, 1943), p. 96.

27.  James 5: 14–18 (Revised Standard Version).

28.  Kelsey, *Healing and Christianity,* chap. 7.

29.  John E. Large, *The Ministry of Healing* (New York: Morehouse–Gorham, 1959), pp. 72–74.

30.  Kelsey, *Healing and Christianity,* p. 201.

31.  H.B. Porter, "The Origin of the Medieval Rite for Anointing the Sick or Dying," *Journal of Theological Studies* 7 (1956): 211–25.

32.  Kelsey, *Healing and Christianity,* chap. 8.

33.  Erwin H. Ackerknecht, *Therapeutics: From the Primitives to the 20th Century* (New York: Hafner Press, 1973), p. 45.

34.  Mary Risley, *House of Healing: The Story of the Hospital* (Garden City, N.Y.: Doubleday, 1961), chaps. 7, 8.

35.  Kelsey, *Healing and Christianity,* pp. 22–27.

36.  Wade H. Boggs, *Faith Healing and the Christian Faith* (Richmond, Va.: John Knox Press, 1956), is a good presentation of this point of view from an admittedly Calvinist perspective.

37.  Ruth Cranston, *The Miracle of Lourdes* (New York: McGraw-Hill, 1955); also Frank, *Persuasion and Healing,* pp. 53–59; Large, *Ministry of Healing,* pp. 119–53.

38.  Mary Baker Eddy, *Science and Health* (Boston: First Church of Christ, Scientist, 1971; first published 1875).

39.  Ahlstrom, *Religious History of the American People,* pp. 819–24; Rene Laurentin, *Catholic Pentecostalism* (Garden City, N.Y.: Doubleday, 1978), pp. 21–24.

40.  David Edwin Harrell, *All Things Are Possible: The Healing and Charismatic Revivals in Modern America* (Bloomington, Ind.: Indiana University Press, 1975).

41.  Harrell, *All Things Are Possible,* pp. 99–100.

42.  Boggs, *Faith Healing.*

43.  Church of England, *Church's Ministry of Healing*, p. 50.

44.  Francis MacNutt, *Healing* (Notre Dame, Ind.: Ave Maria Press, 1974), p. 72.

45.  See Also Kelsey, *Healing and Christianity*, pp. 239-40; and Large, *Ministry of Healing*, pp. 7-9.

46.  Harrell, *All Things Are Possible*, pp. 225-33.

47.  Charles S. Braden, "Study of Spiritual Healing in the Churches," *Pastoral Psychology* 5 (1954): 9-15.

48.  Meredith McGuire, "Health and Holiness: 'Faith Healing' among Catholic Pentecostals," paper presented to the Society for the Scientific Study of Religion, 1978, mimeo.

49.  Arthur Kleinman, "Medicine's Symbolic Reality," *Inquiry* 16 (1973): 206-13.

50.  United Presbyterian Church in the U.S.A., *The Relation of Christian Faith to Health*, 1960; United Lutheran Church in America, *Anointing and Healing: Statement*, 1962; American Lutheran Church, *Christian Faith and the Ministry of Healing*, 1965; Church of Canada, *Handbook on the Healing Ministry of the Church, Report of the Bishop of Toronto's Commission on the Church's Ministry of Healing*, 1968.

51.  Fox, *Church's Ministry of Healing*, chaps. 7, 8.

52.  August Hollingshead and F.C. Redlich, *Social Class and Mental Illness* (New York: John Wiley & Sons, 1958).

53.  Gerald Gurin, Joseph Veroff, and Sheila Feld, *Americans View Their Mental Health* (New York: Basic Books, 1960).

54.  Kenneth C. Haugk, "Unique Contributions of Churches and Clergy to Community Mental Health," *Community Mental Health* 12 (1976): 20-28.

55.  E. Mansell Pattison, "Systems of Pastoral Care," *Journal of Pastoral Care* 26 (1972): 2-14.

56.  Agnes Sanford, *The Healing Light* (Plainfield, N.J.: Logos International, 1976; first published 1947), chap. 14.

57.  Kelsey, *Healing and Christianity*, p. 141.

58.  MacNutt, *Healing*, p. 80.

59.  Richardson, "Spiritual Healing," pp. 206-16.

60.  Kenneth L. Vaux, *This Mortal Coil* (San Francisco: Harper & Row, 1978), p. 37.

61.  MacNutt, *Healing*, p. 86.

62.  John Pitts, *Faith Healing: Fact or Fiction?* (New York: Hawthorn Books, 1961), p. 145.

63.  Richardson, "Spiritual Healing," p. 180.

64.  Bernard Grad, "Some Biological Effects of the 'Laying On of Hands,'" *Journal of Pastoral Counseling* 6 (1971-72): 38-41; Delores Krieger,

"Therapeutic Touch: The Imprimatur of Nursing," *American Journal of Nursing* 75 (1975): 784–87.

65. Lee Hancock, Central Presbyterian Church, New York, personal communication.
66. Kelsey, *Healing and Christianity*, p. 353.
67. Porter, "Origin of Anointing the Sick," p. 221.
68. MacNutt, *Healing*, pp. 276–78.
69. Kathryn Kuhlman, *I Believe in Miracles* (Old Tappan, N.J.: Fleming H. Revell, 1976).
70. Harrell, *All Things Are Possible.*
71. Sanford, *Healing Light.*
72. Ruth Carter Stapleton, *The Experience of Inner Healing* (New York: Bantam Books, 1977).
73. Emily Gardiner Neal, *God Can Heal You Now* (Englewood Cliffs, N.J.: Prentice-Hall, 1958).
74. First-person accounts of the events of that weekend and the early days of the renewal can be found in Kevin and Dorothy Ranaghan, *Catholic Pentecostals* (Paramus, N.J.: Paulist Press, 1969).
75. Laurentin, *Catholic Pentecostalism*, pp. 16–17.
76. Ranaghan and Ranaghan, *Catholic Pentecostals,* mention healing only occasionally. Edward D. O'Connor, *The Pentecostal Movement in the Catholic Church* (Notre Dame, Ind.: Ave Maria Press, 1971), devotes two pages to it.
77. O'Connor, *Pentecostal Movement,* p. 163.
78. Mary Ann Jahr, "A Turning Point," *New Covenant* 4 (1974): 4–7.
79. "Healing Testimonies from the 1974 International Conference on the Catholic Charismatic Renewal," *New Covenant* 4 (1975): 18–20; Laurentin, *Catholic Pentecostalism*, pp. 117–21.
80. Especially MacNutt, *Healing,* but also Michael Scanlan, *Inner Healing* (New York: Paulist Press, 1974); Matthew Linn and Dennis Linn, *Healing of Memories* (Paramus, N.J.: Paulist Press, 1974).
81. Meredith McGuire, "Toward a Sociological Interpretation of the 'Catholic Pentecostal' Movement," *Review of Religious Research* 16 (1975): 94–104.
82. *1979/80 International Directory of Catholic Charismatic Prayer Groups* and *Prayer Group Directory Supplement 1980* (South Bend, Ind.: Servant Publications, 1980).
83. Michael I. Harrison, "Sources of Recruitment to Catholic Pentecostalism," *Journal for the Scientific Study of Religion* 13 (1972): 49–64.
84. McGuire, "Toward a Sociological Interpretation," p. 96.
85. Ibid., p. 97; Harrison, "Sources of Recruitment," p. 52.

86. Ranaghan and Ranaghan, *Catholic Pentecostals,* pp. 167–69; Francis MacNutt, *The Power to Heal* (Notre Dame, Ind.: Ave Maria Press, 1977), pp. 103–7.

87. MacNutt, *Power to Heal,* p. 91.

88. Laurentin, *Catholic Pentecostalism,* p. 31.

89. Ibid., p. 154.

90. McGuire, "Health and Holiness."

91. Ibid., p. 19.

92. MacNutt, *Healing,* pp. 161–63.

93. MacNutt, *Power to Heal,* Introduction, chaps. 10, 13.

94. McGuire, Health and Holiness," p. 13.

95. Ibid., pp. 15–16.

96. Ibid., p. 17.

97. Ibid., pp. 18–19.

98. Luke 9: 43–46.

99. MacNutt, *Healing,* chap. 14.

100. Ibid., chap. 13.

101. Scanlan, *Inner Healing,* p. 12.

102. Linn and Linn, *Healing of Memories.*

103. Thomas J. Chordas and Steven Jay Gross, "The Healing of Memories: Psychotherapeutic Ritual among Catholic Pentecostals," *The Journal of Pastoral Care* 30 (1976): 245–57.

104. See *The Journal of Religion and Health,* for example.

105. MacNutt, *Healing,* chap. 12.

106. See, for example, Matt. 8: 28–32.

107. MacNutt, *Healing,* chap. 15.

108. Chordas and Gross, "Healing of Memories," p. 247.

109. McGuire, "Health and Holiness," pp. 2–3.

110. The story in Appendix B of MacNutt, *Power to Heal,* pp. 237–43, is a good example.

111. Chordas and Gross, "Healing of Memories."

112. MacNutt, *Power to Heal,* pp. 39–45.

113. Ibid., chap. 3.

114. Laurentin, *Catholic Pentecostalism,* p. 35.

115. Ibid., chap. 4.

116. MacNutt, *Power to Heal,* p. 42.

117. MacNutt, *Healing,* pp. 276–85.

118. Ibid., pp. 285–90.

119. George W. Kosicki, "The Healing Power of the Eucharist," *New Covenant,* vol. 4 (1974), pp. 12–15.

120. McGuire, "Toward a Sociological Interpretation," p. 100.

121.  McGuire, "Health and Holiness."
122.  MacNutt, *Power to Heal*, p. 28.
123.  George Martin, "Doctors, Medicine, and Divine Healing," *New Covenant* 7 (1977): 24–26.
124.  MacNutt, *Power to Heal*, pp. 58–59.
125.  McGuire, "Toward a Sociological Interpretation," p. 100.
126.  Ibid., p. 95; Harrison, "Sources of Recruitment," p. 56.
127.  Ibid.
128.  McGuire, "Toward a Sociological Interpretation," p. 101.

# 4 COMMUNITY GROUPS AND MUTUAL AID

There are countless numbers and types of groups of lay people in American communities organized around health issues. Their organizational structures may range from the loosely connected lay referral network of a city neighborhood to the sophisticated national organization of Alcoholics Anonymous, the oldest of the mutual aid groups. Obviously there are too many kinds of groups to be enumerated here. A more modest attempt is made to describe three general categories of groups organized around health issues: the lay referral and help-giving resources of the local neighborhood, which may have certain ethnic or cultural characteristics; the mutual aid or self-help group, whose numbers have been growing at an astounding rate; and volunteer organizations, especially those that use some form of peer counseling. The chapter concludes with a closer look at one new type of volunteer organization, the rape crisis center.

Unlike the family and the church, the subjects of the two previous chapters, these groups are more obviously part of the health resources of our society. Because health care in one form or another is the reason these groups exist, they tend to be more visible and less taken for granted. They are also more amenable to research, to which the small army of social scientists now studying mutual aid groups and hotlines can attest.

Also unlike the family and the church, these groups tend to appear and disappear in response to social conditions that are continually changing. In fact, one of the most important themes of this chapter is the role of these groups in initiating and responding to social change. The fact that these groups are small and indigenously organized, and indeed may not even be aware of the existence of other, very similar groups, makes their pervasiveness in our society quite remarkable. Some of the social conditions to which they are responding have already been examined; the shift from infectious to chronic disease, the widespread criticism of the medical profession, the rising costs of medical care, all have contributed to the extraordinary proliferation of these groups in contemporary society. In effect, these groups provide an accurate measure of the kinds of health problems people feel are not being adequately addressed by anyone else. These social institutions are being spontaneously generated in the cracks and gaps of the professional and nonprofessional health care system.

The historical specificity of some of these groups to our own times should not obscure the continuous existence in our history of lay health organizations. The novelty of some of these groups simply underscores the ingenuity of small-scale social organization. On the other hand, some others are repeating patterns of groups that existed in the nineteenth century and earlier. The point is that lay health organizations are continually appearing and disappearing, arising to fill the needs of a community, existing as long as they are useful, and then disbanding when they have fulfilled their purpose. Unlike bureaucratic or professional structures, which may be maintained with nothing but inertia, lay health organizations rarely outlive their usefulness. People do not continue to volunteer their time to projects that they consider worthless, that seem ineffectual, or that are not personally fulfilling. It is almost as if such groups have a built-in ability to destroy themselves when they cease to be relevant to the needs of their community. This is not meant to imply that such groups are inherently unstable and short-lived. The long record of steady growth of Alcoholics Anonymous shows that, where there are continuing needs for the support a group can give and that group really provides that support, it can continue indefinitely, long past the participation of the original group members.

Health issues have always been a focus of formal and informal social organization in our society. However unique these organizations may seem, voluntary associations concerned with health have a long history in our society. Though health problems have certainly changed, the political, social, and psychological motivations for the formation of these groups in our own time mirror to a remarkable extent the forces at work in earlier periods of our history, particularly during the nineteenth century.

The earliest examples of what we would call voluntary associations mentioned in the literature are the Friendly Societies of seventeenth-century Britain. These were groups of working men who pooled part of their resources to give aid to one another in times of sickness and death. By paying one shilling per quarter, a workman and his family could claim the following benefits: (1) free treatment and prescriptions by a physician in time of sickness; (2) free setting of broken bones by a surgeon; (3) subsistence pay during times of the workman's disability; and (4) free burial for workmen and pensions for the widow.[1] Such societies began in industrialized urban areas of Britain and were always more common there than in rural areas. They did become very widespread, however, and by 1900 there were an estimated 27,000 in existence.[2] These societies were notorious for spending the contributions of their members on drink, but their steady growth over two centuries testifies to the fact that their members at least received an important benefit in the social life the group afforded.[3] They also became quite diversified, so that their services included housing, farm cooperatives, loans, and workmen's compensation. But the original impetus for organization was for the protection of members against the economic effects of sickness and death in a newly industrialized society where one's labor was all one had to sell.

The American health reform movement of the nineteenth century can also be seen, at least in part, as a response to the pains of industrialization. The origin of this movement is traced to Sylvester Graham, a Pennsylvanian who began his career as a Methodist clergyman, became a temperance lecturer, and then expanded his denunciations of alcohol to include tea, coffee, tobacco, and meat.[4] Graham gave lectures throughout the Northeast on personal hygiene, vegetarianism (emphasizing whole wheat products), exercise, bathing, and fresh air. His doctrine of good health habits had a strongly moral tone to it; personal salvation could only be achieved by right living.

His lectures soon spawned groups of right-livers, some of whom had regular meetings to discuss health topics. One group began living together in a boardinghouse in New York in 1833 and eating a strict Graham diet. The first health reform association was formed in Boston in 1837 by a group of Graham followers and Dr. William Alcott, another strong advocate of health and hygiene. The American Physiological Society, as it was called, had as its goal the diffusion of such "plain and practical information . . . as may tend to promote . . . the health and longevity of the whole human family."[5] It also held monthly conferences at which guest lecturers spoke on health and related topics, such as anatomy, dress reform, and sexual hygiene. The society maintained a store in Boston where fresh fruits, vegetables, and whole wheat flour were sold, and published several journals for the education of the public.

The people who belonged to these groups tended to belong to other social reform groups as well—the men living in the Graham boardinghouse in New York were also known as temperance reformers and abolitionists. The women who joined the Ladies' Physiological Societies were early feminists. These women, in fact, constituted a very important part of the health reform movement, and several emerged as its leaders, in particular Mary Gove Nichols and Marie Louise Shew.[6] Health reformers emphasized the wife and mother's role in promoting the physical, moral, and spiritual health of her family, and for this she needed education. The growth of the Ladies' Physiological Societies, with chapters all over New England and the Midwest, was in itself a sort of women's rights movement in a day in which middle-class women rarely spoke to public groups. The appeal of these health reform associations for these women may well lie in the fact that women were undergoing far-reaching changes in their roles as a result of industrialization. Health reform may have seemed a way to reinstitute the stability of the home and to reinforce the woman's importance in it. The rights these women were fighting for seem minimal by today's standards: the right to dress without corsets and stays, the right to an education, and later the right to vote.

The health reform movement reached its apex in the 1860s in the work of Dr. D. H. Trall, but it had by this time become more commercial and professionalized. Trall's "hygienic institute" in New York City offered water cure therapy, diet, exercise, and electrical treatment and was firmly opposed to the use of drugs and the regular practice of medicine. In effect, he joined a "natural" therapeutic system to the health promotion strategies of the health reformers and came up with a complete alternative to the regular medicine of the day.[7]

Much like today's mutual aid groups, the health reform movement benefited primarily its own members by emphasizing the value of personal control in health. It located the source of ill health in the evil habits of individuals: intemperance, gluttony, sloth, vanity. The health reformers felt that these habits could be changed, through education and effort, by any person who wanted to try. Individual health was clearly a matter of personal responsibility. The individualism of this secular health religion had a strong Protestant heritage.

But at another level the health reform movement, whose individualistic concerns ignored the effects of widespread social conditions, can also be seen as a response to industrialization. Not only was it an attempt by individuals and families to overcome the social disorder brought by the industrialization of the cities, but it was also a response to what might be called the industrialization of the medical profession. Just like the medical sects—the Thomsonians and the homeopaths—of which it was a contemporary, the health reform movement sought to make therapeutic medicine milder, simpler, and easier to bear than the heroic therapy of bleeding and purging against which they all were rebelling. All sought natural remedies for prevention and cure—herbs, vegetarian diet, water therapy—and abhorred the use of tools (for bloodletting) and chemicals (for purging the system).[8] Such groups as these, which are organized primarily for the benefit of their own members, are forebears of the contemporary mutual aid group.

But there is also a strong tradition in this country of lay health organizations made up of volunteers whose only personal benefit is the fulfillment of helping others less fortunate than themselves. Beginning in the 1830s during the period of early industrialization and Jacksonian democracy, private philanthropists and volunteers established institutions for the insane and mentally handicapped, rescuing many from the jails and poorhouses where they had been left.[9] These often became problems in themselves, however, as the reformer Dorothea Dix made public in her investigation of insane asylums in Massachusetts. The Civil War saw the establishment of the United States Sanitary Commission, a group of male and female volunteers who nursed the wounded, sick, and dying soldiers in the Union army camps. The experience gained by these volunteers was put to good use when the war was over. They focused their attention on the deplorable conditions in municipal hospitals and almshouses. Middle-class women, in particular, took the leadership of these reform-minded volunteers and formed associations such as the New York State Charities Aid Association.[10] The plan of the Charities Aid Association to improve conditions at Bellevue Hospital and other urban institutions may have been extremely naive, based on the belief that the very presence of women in these places would effect reform. But they did bring many abuses to public attention. They also founded the Bellevue School of Nursing to train nurses in the sanitary care of the sick.

The women reformers who established settlement houses, such as Jane Addams in Chicago and Lillian Wald in New York, had special interests in health care, particularly for women and children. They worked closely with local governments to operate baby health stations where mothers could obtain cheap, fresh milk for their babies and the advice of public health nurses on the care of their children. The settlement house workers maintained a broad agenda of social-political reform based on their early epidemiological investigations into the causes of infant mortality, concluding that the high rates in cities were a result of the environmental conditions of poverty, crowding, poor sanitation, and poor nutrition.[11]

Those associations known as our national voluntary health organizations, which usually concern themselves with a specific disease, began to be founded at the turn of the century. The oldest is the National Tuberculosis Association, founded in 1904 by Dr. Lawrence Flick, who used women volunteers to distribute educational pamphlets and collect money by selling Christmas seals for a penny apiece.[12] Other volunteer organizations soon formed to raise money for heart disease, cancer, arthritis, polio, muscular dystrophy, and many others. Funds were divided between treatment of those who had the disease, research into its causes, prevention, cure, and public education. Perhaps the most successful research funded in this way was the work done by Dr. Jonas Salk at the University of Pittsburgh, which led to the development of a vaccine for polio in 1955.[13]

Today these associations are large, complex institutions with enormous budgets. Most have become rather highly professionalized, though many require a certain percentage of laymen on their decision-making boards. Even their fund raising has become professionalized to a certain extent by television entertainers but ultimately it depends on the volunteered time and effort of thousands of Americans.

More attention will be given later to the new roles of volunteers who do more than raise money. These new forms of volunteering are more like those much earlier in our history, when men and women helped other people directly, though the services offered today are more likely to be peer counseling than dressing battle wounds.

One important point has not yet been made. All these voluntary associations, including social reform groups, health reform groups, national voluntary health organizations, networks, volunteer-staffed hotlines and crisis centers, and mutual aid groups, are the products of a democratic society. Whether such groups benefit themselves or others, anyone is free to join or to start his own group. Only in a society where people are free to associate as they see fit and to organize around the issues that seem most pressing to them could such a diversity of groups appear and flourish.

## KINSHIP AND FRIENDSHIP NETWORKS

As we have seen, the preponderance of health and medical care is self-provided by the individual or the immediate family. An important aspect of this service is interpreting symptoms and deciding what action to take, including doing nothing. Clearly, culture and social class affect the decision and subsequent care behavior. But of equal importance in influencing health actions is the process of decision making within the social context of family and community. Parents do make decisions on behalf of children, and adults similarly rely on others to help define the health situation and advise on a course of action. Eliot Freidson, in his classic work *Patients' View of Medical Practice,* was the first to describe this process as a lay referral system that operates within a definable structure. The lay referral structure denotes a pathway of using informal "consultants" in a progressive sequence leading toward increasingly "more select, distinct authoritative persons until the 'professional' is reached. It is a network of referrals in that consultants not only diagnose and prescribe but also make referrals."[14] As Freidson observed in his 1961 study of subscribers to a prepaid group practice plan, social class and culture shape the lay referral system and structure by reflecting social/cultural variations in the meaning of illness, level of medical (allopathic) sophistication, familiarity with professional resources, and relationship with health professionals, especially physicians.

Since Freidson's early work, mainstream research on the lay referral system has focused heavily on its complicity in causing delays in seeking professional care, not following professional advice, or failure to seek professional help altogether. Recently, however, there is a more positive interest in the lay referral as a mediating force (as a buffer analogous to the contribution of "second opinions" in professional decisions), as a social support resource, and as a substantial health care resource. We are beginning to appreciate lay referral as an integral part of the health coping system that influences the when, who, what, and how of medical care. At the same time, a renewed interest in social networks as moderators of stress, producers of help, and transmitters of information and innovation has deepened our appreciation of the health care contribution of nonprofessional social resources. There are, to be sure, large theoretical and methodological problems in achieving a secure basis for predicting how these social networks function and in precisely measuring their effects. Nevertheless, studies under way will begin to fill in the picture of health care as a total social resource. Health organizational theory, economic modeling, resources allocation, and, indeed, the full sweep of health planning will now have available a powerful corrective to the present professional construction of health care. At last the general shape of the lay health resource is emerging, and an exciting alternative to present professional systems research is apparent.

It is accepted as conventional wisdom that the American family has become an atomized and isolated social unit, bearing little resemblance to the extended family of yesteryear. We view with alarm the disintegration of the nuclear family and the erosion of extended families. Much of our belief stems from the physical evidence of the family domiciliary configuration of parents and children, absent grandparents, in-laws, or other relatives sharing the same board. We count the single-family dwellings and the single-parent families as loners, estranged for various reasons (economic, psychological) that the modern world engenders. Evidence that disputes this perspective has been available for nearly three decades; yet the commitment to an atomistic, nuclear perspective on the family has been overwhelming. Marvin Sussman, in a cogent review appearing in 1959, concluded:

> The answer to the question "The Isolated Nuclear Family, 1959: Fact or Fiction?" is, mostly fiction. It is suggested that kin ties, particularly intergenerational ones, have far more significance than we have been led to believe in the life processes of the urban family. While these kin ties are by no means replicate [sic] the 1890 model, the 1959 neolocal nuclear family is not completely atomistic but closely integrated within a network of mutual assistance and activity which can be described as an independent kin family system.[15]

Telephone and convenient transportation appear to be effective compensation for the loss of close geographic proximity of kin. Thus the kinship network continues to be a viable helping resource. In referring to his study of kin and family relationships in Cleveland, Sussman reported that "practically all families (100 percent of the middle class and 92.5 percent of the working class) were considered to be actively involved in a network of inter-familial help by virtue of giving or receiving one or more items of assistance . . . within a one month period."[16] At the very least, on the basis of the data in hand, we are compelled to take a closer look at the kin (and friendship) network as it exists in its contemporary modalities and functions.

Overcoming geographic separation, communication among family members continues to provide mutual exchange of information and advice. This is a particularly important contribution when family members face decisions in which experience interpreted through commonly held values is critical. The decision to seek professional health assistance and managing the assistance received are two examples. The health care experience of American Gypsies is a case in point. One might expect on the basis of their poverty and minority status, often compounded by language differences and peripatetic life-styles, that American Gypsies would be at least as badly served by the health system as the mainstream minority poor. But apparently this is not true. In his research on urban Gypsies, Jeffrey

Salloway found several mitigating aspects of Gypsy culture and social structure that resulted in an effective pattern of use of health care:

> The characteristics which may make the Gypsies better consumers of medical care than other such groups are their willingness to reject the entire medical system because of one or more bad experiences, their inherent mobility, their willingness to "shop" for good services, and their ability to locate such services through their extensive networks.[17]

The extended family and friendship network is the integral core of Gypsy life. Individuals are not alone in pursuit of health care and are literally surrounded with vigilant kith and kin during the care process. A blank check of trust is never offered the professional care provider. Care is a fully shared experience in which nothing is taken for granted, in which the diagnosis and treatment procedures are mediated by family and friends to ensure that options, consequences, and costs are known. Gypsies do not expect a break; indeed, they are constantly alert to the presence of bias in their care. In effect, their expectations are realistic, and the strategy of protecting one another is appropriate and apparently effective.

Salloway, impressed by the selectivity and streetwise approach to medical care so visible among the Gypsies, speculated that nonuse of services by disadvantaged groups in effect forms a socially based judgment, rational and purposeful, of the quality of care. The Gypsy network acts to test the efficacy of the care given and offers the individual the support necessary to reject care and go elsewhere.

The kinship and friendship support system of the American urban Gypsy is a dramatic but nonetheless useful example to sharpen our awareness of comparable functions in mainstream society. At the level of personal experience, there is an implicit acceptance of the day-to-day contribution of extended family and friends in support of health and welfare. But our awareness of this resource as such has been obscured by the ethic of professional services as the esteemed and legitimate strategy for care and a corollary depreciation of amateurism in human services. Recent social research seeking to define and predict the caring role of family and friends is beginning to correct this bias. For example, a study by Allan Horwitz of psychiatric help seeking tells us that a sharing, mutually supportive husband-wife relationship reduces the need for help from extended family and friends when a psychiatric problem arises.[18] But since only 21 percent of married couples he studied provided such support, the extended family and friendship network became an important basic resource for these nuclear families.

It is such parsing of the network that can define its dimensions and operating laws and rationalize empirical data in ways useful for promoting development of the network resource. But in reviewing myriad studies of networks, one is struck by the lack of a standard nomenclature and wide variations in study populations and research methods. Since Karen Petersen's plea for greater comparability, a decade has passed with little noticeable improvement.[19] A collage-like impression of networks as a health resource is the result. On the other hand, where some specific need to know arises, particularly with a sense of perceived urgency (that is, it is critical for health or economic effects) there has been considerably more in-depth and linked research. The practical reasons for getting a handle on the contributions of networks to professional health care are the most obvious cases in point. How people find their way into the health care system, the question of lay referral, is the specific example of network function that has received concerted attention. Research benefits here can go directly to several longstanding goals of public health, such as reducing delay in seeking professional help and achieving greater efficiency of health services use. Certainly these and similar goals are criticized as self-seeking, to perpetuate and expand professional control of the lay health resource.[20] Nevertheless, the appeal of research on this aspect of helping networks[21] —whether pure or prurient—appears to be the major item of research interest selected from a wide menu of possibilities.[22] There remain gaps in our knowledge of the entire system of health care decisions and actions, the branching design of lay health care activity. As noted, research fragments on the health implications of networks are more productive of hypotheses than of operational models. There are teasing insights into the role of extended family and friends. An example is a study of men who suffered a first myocardial infarction and the perceived level of help they received from extended family and friends. In this study by Sydney Croog, Alberta Lipson, and Sol Levine, there was a careful analysis of attributes associated with perceived degrees of support provided by these nonprofessional resources, including age of patients, education, social class, social interaction level, ethnic origins, and level of the patient's need.[23] Croog and his colleagues also looked at the types of help provided by extended family as differentiated from "outside" sources of neighbors and friends. They concluded that help received from neighbors and friends carried substantial integrity as a distinct resource supplementary to, rather than compensatory for, help received from the family. Most important, the findings of this study failed to support the conventional views that (1) the nuclear family is structurally isolated (at least in time of critical need) and (2) the help functions of family and friends are transferred to professional care givers to a significant extent.[24]

Extended family and friends as care-giving support resources will probably undergo more detailed scrutiny with regard to characteristics of services performed and the phasing of those services. How severe a crisis draws in family or precludes friends? When do various elements of the caring network begin their involvement, and how long can they be counted on? Are there aspects of certain health problems that are too intimate or too stigmatizing or too draining to attract one or another sector of the network care-giving resource? What are the elements of the care recipient–network dyad that would predict the greatest benefits to *both* the recipient and the network?

How can we approach answers to these and related questions on networks as health and health care productive systems? A most convenient strategy simply would be to apply utilization review and accounting methods now used to assess the productivity of the professional care system. But it is clear that substantial differences in ethic and enterprise between the lay care network and a professional care system would preclude such an application. The lay network is a *mutual* system in which the roles of providers and recipient are fluid, and role exchanges are an integral part of measuring the efficacy, particularly the efficiency, of the network system. This is in contrast to the sharply differentiated roles of provider and consumer in the professional service domain. Here *role predictability* becomes a central measure of efficacy.

The lay care network, in contrast to the professional system, is governed by laws of demand and effective demand (supply) that are not subject to the usual constraints of the market (capital) economy and its regulation by professional monopolies or government standards. There are, therefore, none of the benchmarks or usual evidences of service that are available in commercial-professional transactions.

The help seeker's criteria for tapping network resources for diagnosis, treatment, continuing care, or social support need not include items useful in determining cultural and social compatibility, which are implicit in criteria applied to seeking professional services. Will the physician understand me, know my concerns and preferences, and honor them? This question and the attendant criteria for judging are unnecessary in the network context. On the other hand, we have come to expect that the network resource offers powerful benefits in its interactional properties. In this context, our judgment of the network is in terms of the support provided, such as "nourishment to self-esteem, normative affirmation, dependency relatedness, clarification of expectations if needed, and the discharge of disturbing affects, etc."[25]

Other discrepancies of function and relationship cause us to conclude that it is not feasible or relevant to account for the health contributions of networks as we account for the process and outcomes of professional care. As a mutual social system, accountability for network effects must be both multidimensional (provide support, provide care, provide protection) and multilateral (benefit individuals as well as community). Traditional approaches to defining, predicting, and evaluating the essentially dyadic, one-dimensional, and unilateral interaction of patient and care giver have, in fact, not held much appeal for researchers working on lay health care networks. Indeed, the theoretical framework for measuring network health care functions appears to be derived from the earlier (and still dominant) interest in networks as social support systems. The medical care function of networks is merely identified as one among several attributes of network support. The matrix of observations required to account for network health care functions must allow us to differentiate care from caring *not* as product versus process, but with both having distinct effects on health. In the professional construction of health care, caring is an aspect of service delivery; in the network construction of health care, it is a specific contribution to protecting, to mediating between the individual and the threat of disease and iatrogenic hazards.

Depending on what function we are talking about, accounting for network contributions to health presents different problems. Perhaps the least problematic in this regard are the networks' roles in facilitating access to professional services (lay referral) and in the direct provision of health care. Regarding their referral role, we are well down the road of describing the interactional design and the variations that are related to demographic characteristics of those involved in the interaction. Such analyses serve to destroy the myth of an atomistic society in health decision making and are useful in arguing the case for declassifying professional and evaluative information, which can enhance the effectiveness of the lay referral system.[26] Accounting for the care-giving functions of networks, while far from avoiding the research biases introduced by observing only those activities defined against professional criteria, is still largely a matter of developing a feasible nonprofessional technology to record lay-defined health activities.

In contrast to these functions of networks, those of providing support and mediation to prevent disease or reduce its negative sequelae are the least understood. It is possible that clarification of these functions will be professionally or even politically uninteresting to those committed to explanations of disease as rooted either in biological man or in economic man, two sectors of the human condition immediately (and therefore appealingly) available to professional or political preventive intervention. Indeed, the contribution of networks to reducing mortality is a consequence or byproduct of social integration, not an outcome of purposeful action. It is the *existence* of network links that prevents and protects. Thus there is no apparent basis for manipulation beyond the nurturance of social interaction. Although recognized as a powerful factor associated with lower mortality independent of the usual predicters of mortality (demographic status and personal health habits), the specific mechanisms involved in network effects on mortality are still matters of speculation. Lisa Berkman and S. Leonard Syme, for example, offer three hypotheses: (1) that there is an association between isolation and poor health practices; (2) that isolation contributes to depression or ability to cope; and (3) that social isolation causes physiologic changes that in turn increase susceptibility to disease.[27] Evidence presented by the Berkman and Syme study, together with many previous studies on the positive relation of social integration to reduced morbidity and mortality reviewed in Chapter 1, could become the basis for research that could help define preventive strategies that may become an integral part of social development.

### Mutual Aid Groups

Mediating structures in health are pervasive in our daily lives. They are virtually synonymous with social life, an essential element of the plasma that nourishes the growth, character, and safety of the human group. The first and most profoundly pervasive and accessible level of helping is the natural social structure itself: families, friends, and neighborhoods. At a more purposive level, such voluntary associations as unions and social clubs serve to preserve and promote the health of their members, though not necessarily (or usually) by plan or design. And finally there is the level of social, nonprofessional resources organized with the expressed intent of providing direct and immediate health benefits for their members: mutual aid or self-help groups.

Mutual aid groups in America have multiplied during the four decades since the founding of Alcoholics Anonymous. Several excellent texts have traced their emergence, their morphology, their functions, and their benefits as well as their possible social costs. Our purpose here is to clarify the salient aspects of mutual aid groups as powerful mediating structures, particularly as they address health needs.

Alfred Katz offers a simple and generic definition of mutual aid as "the taking and giving of help to one another in natural or specially-created social groups and networks"[28] This formulation is a particularly appropriate way to identify a social phenomenon that is rooted in so many dimensions of human experience and needs. Attempts to codify mutual aid groups are the best testimony to their diversity. Morphologies have been proposed that share a similar pool of observations yet organize this information in somewhat different ways. As Katz noted, we are still "in a Linnaean phase of collecting representative types and developing a nomenclature for them."[29] Katz, whose work is most extensively available in the literature on self-help, suggests four clusters of mutual aid groups around their primary focus and a fifth cluster in which there does not seem to be a single dominant focus:

1. Groups that focus primarily on self-fulfillment or personal growth (for example, Recovery, Inc.);

2. Groups that focus primarily on social advocacy (for example, the Committee for the Rights of the Disabled);
3. Groups whose primary focus is to create alternative patterns for living (gay rights' and women's liberation groups);
4. Outcast havens, or "rock-bottom" groups, which provide a refuge for desperate people who are seeking protection from the pressures of life and society (for example, X-Kalay Foundation in Canada).[30]

A typology of mutual aid groups with a dominant health interest is offered by Alan Gartner and Frank Riessman.[31] They cite four central categories: (1) rehabilitative (concerned with adjustment to a new situation, such as stroke, mastectomy); (2) behavior modification (examples include control of alcohol consumption, drugs, smoking); (3) primary care for chronic disease (coping and caring strategies are learned); and (4) preventive and case finding (people with a common interest in organizing community efforts to achieve early detection of, for example, hypertension). Other experienced observers of mutual aid health-oriented groups are content merely to emphasize the distinction between true mutual aid groups in health and those "foundation-oriented" groups that emphasize research, public education, fund-raising, and legislation, namely, the major voluntary associations (American Lung Association, American Cancer Society).[32]

"Mutual aid group" is a relatively recent label applied to the contemporary form of a social design that reaches back, in the view of anthropologist Sol Tax, at least as far as the Middle Pleistocene Era in the form of families, hunting parties, and religious congregations.[33] What is new is our further institutionalization of its role and the debate engendered as we try to reconcile the ethic, purpose, and contribution of mutual aid groups with our current belief in (and economic-social commitment to) the world of professional service.

Recognition of the mutual aid group as a ubiquitous and popular social resource in health has drawn attention to the interface implications of mutual aid and professional services. At one level, there is keen interest in operational linkages, particularly in the process of professional referral of patients to mutual aid groups.[34] At another level, policy issues are raised on how mutual aid and lay health initiatives may affect health planning, use of professional resources, and evaluation criteria.[35]

There are an estimated 700,000 to 800,000 mutual aid groups in the United States, which include more than 10 million persons.[36] Some partial breakdowns of membership by problem category are cited, but since there is no general accounting mechanism, it is possible only to extrapolate from data fragments.[37] For some major metropolitan areas, directories of mutual aid groups have been published, but it is clear that the proliferation of groups is so rapid that the reliability of these sources as a census of mutual aid groups is uncertain. An effort to collect and collate information on mutual aid groups is under way on a voluntary basis through several clearinghouses, including the National Self-Help Clearinghouse and other regional and local organizations. These offer some perspective on the substantive range of mutual aid groups and a sense of their wide geographic availability.[38] Although we can glean some idea of the sheer magnitude of the movement from these sources, the question of the relative occurrence of mutual aid as a health strategy among social classes and racial and ethnic groups is still unclear. At least one observer avers that mutual aid groups are a mainstream middle-class phenomenon with less appeal to minorities and the poor.[39] Such a blanket assertion, however, is subject to the bias of the criteria being applied. Given that mutual aid groups are culturally sensitive social forms, it may be that their existence is simply not disclosed when we apply established formats and labels foreign to a given social setting. The appeal (perceived benefits) of mutual aid may be expected to vary among social and cultural groups, thus making projections of its growth very uncertain. For example, mutual aid groups may form in stressed and alienated communities to acquire what Kurt Bock and Rebecca Taylor cite as the "emotional benefits of community" otherwise denied them.[40] It seems to us that there is no valid evidential basis to circumscribe the present and future of mutual aid groups by any cultural or demographic determinants.

Social research on the mutual aid phenomenon is subject to the benefits and liabilities of observing and interpreting events in midstream. We have the opportunity to collect substantial data on the characteristics of mutual aid group membership, processes of formation and dissolution, functions, and outcomes. We can define central issues of interface among groups and between mutual aid and corresponding professional resources. But the dispersion of mutual aid in so many new forms and purposes allows only speculation about its social appeal and impact. The result is an array of opinion that reflects primarily differences in the disciplinary and ideological bias of the observers. However, five aspects of mutual aid are commonly cited and provide testimony of the diverse bases of its appeal in contemporary American society.

*1. The Need for Mutual Aid*    Mutual aid groups are formed in response to a deficit in the professional health care system, including the services of physicians, social workers, rehabilitation counselors, psychologists, occupational and physical therapists, and others. It is clear that the allopathic health care system developed its contemporary perspectives and goals during an era when infectious, acute diseases dominated. The professional ethic was to cure. The technology and institutions of medicine focused on acute disease and the acute exacerbations of chronic disease. Health promotion, disease prevention (with the exception of immunization), and rehabilitation were and remain peripheral concerns of medical care. The lack of interest and disinclination to move beyond the high technology and scientific phase of acute care, most dramatically represented in surgical and radiological interventions, appear to have left a vacuum of services to the chronically ill. These needs are physical, psychological, social, and sometimes political. Whether or not professionals could or should provide these services is debatable on several grounds. It might not be so much a matter of default but a rational consequence of an appropriate division of function. The differentiation of function may reflect real distinctive qualifications and limitations, both technical and economic, of professionals and lay persons. Indeed, as Illich and his colleagues have pointed out, professional resources have already usurped some lay health care prerogatives.[41] For health professionals, they argue, to extend their responsibilities further into chronic disease and disability management would be counterproductive and not in the interests of society. Mutual aid groups have steadfastly rejected professional control in favor of a "don't call us, we'll call you" attitude. Although there is merit in the view that mutual aid groups were formed in response to professional deficits in service, it is certainly manifest now that their contribution has integrity in its own right. What benefits accrue through the mutual aid process, particularly the added values of group solidarity and social support, are unique benefits.[42] Mutual aid also has been a source of health care innovation, so much so that in some instances the health professionals learn from and adopt approaches drawn directly from the lay sector. Stephen Jencks cites "Geiger's Law" with respect to this. "When the counter-culture develops something of value, the establishment rips it off and sells it back."[43]

The need for mutual aid groups to complement professional services and provide substantial independent benefits is recognized by health professionals. Health professionals occasionally have taken the initiative in sponsoring or organizing mutual aid groups and more commonly refer patients to them. This is important to emphasize to establish a balanced perspective on mutual aid groups in health as they play the advocate role. While mutual aid is a powerful mediating resource between the lay patient and the professonal, that is not to say that this relationship is a negative reaction to technical medical values or procedures. Most members of mutual aid groups retain their personal medical care from health professionals while they are active participants in mutual aid. Membership in mutual aid groups, however, allows and may even encourage exploration of nonallopathic strategies in health care. It is not uncommon for mutual aid group members to explore non-Western healing strategies and to honor indigenous remedies derived from their particular culture and traditions. Nor is the essential and crucial deficit filled by mutual aid groups wholly definable in terms of desired services; it is at least equally filling a deficit in the power the patients have to control their health destinies, to make effective choices among options, and to participate actively in their own care.

*2. The Bond of Common Experience*     Members of mutual aid groups in health tend to believe their own experience is a more fruitful asset than professional expertise. There is an obvious bond between people who share a common problem that threatens to disrupt their lives and severely limit their capacity to survive as effective and independent social beings. It simply feels right to consult with others who are experiencing the same personal and social consequences of a disease or disorder. The level of trust is high; one need not be suspicious of the competing motives so often associated with professional care. Open communication among members is easily established without the inhibitions and "psychosemantics" that are often part of the patient-professional relationship.[44] The pooling of experience offers a special corrective to any dominant medical strategy or value system.[a] Members credit each other with being in a uniquely favorable position to perceive their problem in its several dimensions at the same time and in an integrated way. Thus the ideas and methods of self-management reflect a real life quality. Credibility is high, allowing trust to grow not only between members but within the individual as a sense of self-worth.

*3. Reciprocity of Aid*    Mutuality of effort is by definition the unique attribute of the mutual aid group. Participation in a mutual aid group is a process of serving and being served, of teaching and being taught, and of achieving a constructive interdependency. Katz defines this as mutually reinforcing the strengths of all parties.[45] This is in sharp contrast to the unbalanced power relationship of patient and physician, a relationship described by Helen Marieskind and Barbara Ehrenreich as one "in which knowledge is the private property of the provider and gives her or him the power to dominate the less privileged, propertyless patient."[46] Shared knowledge not only results in shared power; it also allows mutual aid members to consider collective action as problems in common become revealed.

*4. Political Potential*    Mutual aid groups are not inherently political. As Bender and Katz have observed, an individual member's discontent is shared with fellow members rather than being "internalized as private agendas."[47] There are, however, wide differences among mutual aid groups with regard to their commitment to mobilizing this group process as a resource for concerted social action with effects beyond the group. The advocacy role can be between members, or it can extend to protecting the rights and interests of the entire class of people with a common health cause. Many factors influence the relative emphasis on personal and social advocacy, but the precise conditions that pertain are not fully understood. Furthermore, a historical explanation may be more useful than an assumption that there is something inherent in a given health problem or

---

a. The exception is the ideologically based group (e.g., Alcoholics Anonymous), which demands allegiance to a set standard of belief and behavior.

the demographic characteristics of a group that would predict the mix of personal versus social advocacy. As a group matures in its mutual understanding of the sociopolitical environment that affects its welfare and as it begins to form networks with similar groups, the potential for political action may come more clearly into focus. Another historical explanation was proposed by Katz and Bender, who noted:

> There is some evidence that groups formed in the wake of the counterculture movement of the late 1960s are more inwardly turning than earlier self-help groups. Consciousness-raising toward self-change in the former— what might be termed the "privatization of need"—contrasts with the social action and political thrust more characteristic of groups in other periods.[48]

The central point here is that mutual aid groups in health, with the exception of the ideologically committed groups (such as Alcoholics Anonymous, and its derivatives, Overeaters Anonymous and Gamblers Anonymous) are not bound to a prescribed social outlook. Groups generate and regenerate their content, modus operandi, and goals, which inevitably reflect current needs and priorities. The social charter that holds the group together is *their* product. If the group ceases to benefit its members as the members perceive these benefits, the mutual aid group destroys itself. This constitutes a pragmatic and efficient system of client accountability, quite distinct from the experience of professional care-giving agencies, which often develop a life of their own regardless of social utility.

*5. Communication within the Group*    Mutual aid groups possess organizational integrity. None of the previous comments should imply that mutual aid groups in health are formless, volatile, or casual. Although many are formed seemingly spontaneously, without benefit or blessing from established health organizations, and are largely lacking the usual bureaucratic forms and rituals, the mutual aid group achieves and maintains a clear, dependable identification for its members. Face-to-face relationships in the typically small (ten-person) group make communications naturally easy and efficient. Indeed, the mutual aid group enjoys the benefits of any small group enterprise, especially the absence of hierarchical structure and the presence of a common value system.

Mutual aid groups meet regularly, designate a minimal leadership structure, and plan programs and resources for each meeting. Most groups depend on word of mouth and modest public service publicity to attract members. There are groups whose members are largely referred by physicians, but for the most part the decision to join is the free choice of the individual. Professionally sponsored mutual aid groups, like those supported by major voluntary health associations, may tend to be somewhat more structured in membership criteria and educational program, and less productive of innovations that differ from the beliefs and values of the professional sponsor. But easy generalizations among or between groups based on sponsorship are on uncertain ground. Many factors affect the modality of the mutual aid group. Disease-specific groups may vary widely in their technological dependency on professionals and the level of their need to establish evidence of their effectiveness, their need for legitimization by the referent health profession, and their need for referrals from professionals.[49] The specific character of the mutual aid group's modality is also influenced by other attributes of its problem focus, such as rehabilitation, behavior modification, mutual primary care, prevention, and case finding.[50] In addition, as Katz noted, their longevity, ideology, and myriad sociocultural factors are influential in shaping the mutual aid group's structure as well as functions.[51]

## Mutual Aid Groups as a Health Service Alternative

There are many views regarding where and how the mutual aid group relates to professional health services. Some perspectives deal with the technical interface, identifying the relative expertise of the lay and professional resource. These views of the relationship define the process (and problems) of achieving optimal cooperation, a productive division of labor, based on an underlying assumption of a shared value system. In this construction, the mutual aid group is seen as an important adjunct to professional services, as a helping extension either through supplementation, by providing unique services not offered routinely by professional care givers, or through providing services previously offered by professionals. Other perspectives on mutual aid as alternative service concentrate on the adversarial nature of the mutual aid–professional relationship. Here the emphasis is on an assumed difference in values related to the definition of the problem, the range of solutions, and priorities. Underlying this view of mutual aid and professional relations as essentially competitive is the notion that the self-help group in health is born out of dissatisfaction with the professional system as being deficient in either services or attitudes. The latter may include unbalanced emphasis on the abnormal state of the patient or subtle but powerful reenforcement of the patient's dependency on professional services. There are no substantial data to form a judgment of which view pertains and, given the diversity of mutual aid groups and their constant flux of purpose and function, it is unlikely that a definitive answer will come soon, if ever.

A major clarification to our understanding of mutual aid as an alternative health service was prepared by James S. Gordon for the final report to the President's Commission on Mental Health.[52] On the basis of personal work experience with alternative health services and research undertaken especially for the Commission, Gordon distilled thirteen "philosophical assumptions, attitudes and practices," which reveal themselves as the most significant contributors to the effectiveness of alternative health services, including mutual aid. Cited specifically in reference to mental health alternative services, they are generally relevant to alternative services responding to a wide spectrum of needs.

They respond to people's problems as those problems are experienced.

They provide services that are immediately accessible with a minimum of waiting and bureaucratic restriction.

They tend to treat their client's problems as signs of change and opportunities for growth rather than symptoms of an illness which must be suppressed.

They treat those who come to them for help as members of families and social systems.

They make use of mental health professionals and the techniques they have developed but depend on non-professionals to deliver most of the primary care.

They regard active participation as a cornerstone of their mental health service program and indeed mental health.

They provide both clients and staff with a supportive and enduring community which transcends the delivery of receipt of a particular service.

They change and expand the work they do to meet the changing needs of their clients.

They address themselves to the economic and social handicaps from which their clients suffer.

They can provide care that is by any standards equal or superior to that offered by traditional mental health centers.

They are in general more economical than the traditional services which their clients might otherwise use.

They have financial problems.

They use their experience in trying to meet people's direct service needs as a basis for advocacy efforts on their clients' behalf.[53]

These characteristics identify integral distinctions between alternative and professional services. They are put forward as a complex of features that explain why as well as how alternative services have been so attractive, have proliferated exponentially, and have apparently been successful in meeting the needs of the participants. One can discern an amalgam of the central theories of mutual aid development: (1) mutual aid is a response to needs not met by formal social institutions; (2) mutual aid provides an alternative to an existing service; (3) mutual aid groups form out of a need for support through and by those with similar problems; and (4) mutual aid groups are another form of social organization (in addition to family, labor unions, fraternal clubs) that meets people's needs for intimacy and affiliation.[54] Clearly these attributes of mutual aid and the theories that rationalize their origins and purpose are not assignable uniformly, or on the basis of any known formula, to all forms of mutual aid. Further, the pragmatism of mutual aid and the optimism that pervades its participants and its advocates provide testimony of benefits but are no substitute for the evidence of effectiveness (absolute and relative) based on standard social research. Of course, the rapid growth of the mutual aid group *is* evidence that needs are being met; the questions remain, *what* needs are being met, what are the relative costs and benefits, how durable and potentiating are the results, and are there counterproductive effects?

An overarching issue is how to proceed to answer those questions; how to design an evaluation scheme that reflects the expectations of participants and the definitions they assign to benefits. Indeed, are mutual aid groups and other forms of alternative health service appropriate for evaluation under the terms usually applied to experimental interventions? We believe there is a serious question of appropriateness, given that mutual aid groups are not experimental but developmental in the context of social change. It is as if we were to attempt to measure the absolute or relative benefits of marriage versus living together. Those who elect one mode of relationship over another may differ substantially, thus obviating comparative evaluation. Participants in mutual aid groups may similarly differ from those who do not use them as well as those who use professional resources. The lack of random assignment, the lack of uniformity among groups with regard to priorities and procedures, and the lack of comparability with professional services of many mutual aid outcomes portend failure for an evaluation based on experimental design. In any case, it is not primarily a question of the relative benefits of mutual aid and professional services. These are not competing modalities as much as complementary ones. Surely there are outcomes in which both could claim an interest, but this does not imply that they assign similar priorities or apply comparable levels of effort or expertise to achieving and maintaining them. The challenge of research on mutual aid appears to be one of measuring relative outcomes among mutual aid strategies themselves. Many of the central benefits of mutual aid, in contrast with professional care, are in the process rather than exclusively or even mainly in disease/disorder management skills. Mutual aid itself is what people seek, the sense of oneness leading to a sense of personal wholeness. Here is a caring environment that nurtures personal control and at the same time demonstrates the potential of communal action. In evaluating the role of mutual aid, it is necessary, therefore, to account for personal benefits (process as well as problem-related skills) and the impact of mutual aid on society, that is, its impact on public attitudes about deviant health status and its contributions to changing professional approaches to health care.

*In Summary*  Mutual aid groups have become a pervasive and diverse social resource in health. They are formed largely out of lay initiatives, and they function under the control of their members. Active participation is the key. Experience is the master teacher, and the equity it provides the group obviates the need for hierarchical structure, accountability mechanisms, or dependency on external resources for financing. Members of mutual aid groups benefit as they contribute both in personal health management and adaptive skills and in affecting social factors that inhibit or enhance the health status of the membership.

There are many theories and unanswered questions about why mutual aid groups form (and have multiplied so rapidly), how they function productively, and the nature of their personal and social impact. Their extraordinary diversity of membership, problems, and styles suggests that we are a good distance from useful generalizations. A breakthrough to understanding mutual aid as a practical health resource and as a social, perhaps even political, phenomenon may emerge from the groups themselves. Mutual aid groups are developing a consciousness of their universality and most assuredly will themselves seek ways to communicate their roles in health and social development.

As participants in the first international congress on mutual aid noted, the sweep of the concept of mutual aid itself offers wide latitude for expression in its social forms and is not limited to one culture or type of political environment.[55] Organizations of welfare mothers in Australia, hypertension clubs in Yugoslavia, relatives of mental patients in Austria, and consciousness raising among children in England were testimony to the utility of the role of mutuality, in the power of the lay collectivity to meet both individual and social health needs.

## THE LAY VOLUNTEER IN COMMUNITY HEALTH

We have described the lay resource in health in ever-widening rings of service, from self-service of the individual and family and mutual service in the context of self-help groups through the contributions of religious organizations to healing. These endogenous resources in health have emerged with little or no reference to the professional care-giving system. They appear out of a social heritage, a common wisdom of pragmatic experience and beliefs. In the modern world, the health technology of lay care giving has drawn on various professional skills and concepts, but these lay activities by and large have remained within their historical social template. Thus an exception to this rule takes on special interest as a portent of changes in the professional service monolith, in its resources, and in its style.

The role of lay people as health volunteers is distinct from their endogenous care-giving roles as family members and friends in two important respects: (1) they are performing a purposeful service function on a stranger-to-stranger basis, and (2) their service role either mimics a counterpart professional role or is an extension of a professional service. Examples, which we will turn to later, are volunteers in suicide prevention, rape crisis control, sex counseling, and cancer counseling programs.

Voluntary service by lay persons constitutes an historical but growing and pervasive mediating structure in health. They represent a contemporary form of organized volunteerism in health that evolved from earlier forms of community health action. Richard Carter, in an evenhanded critique of voluntary health associations in the United States, traces the social, religious, economic, and political roots of "charitable good works," which eventually become institutionalized in the modern form of voluntary health associations.[56] Such organizations as the American Lung Association, the American Cancer Society, and the American Heart Association now constitute a major component of the American health care "system."[57] With affiliates at the local and state levels, voluntary health organizations perform services in support of public and professional education related to a specific disease or disability, development of relevant health care services, and the encouragement of disease-specific research. They often lobby for special-interest legislation and not infrequently have supplied public health functions to communities unable to support an official health agency.

Established voluntary associations are an important conduit for lay participation in community service, but they are clearly disciplined bureaucracies where volunteers work on behalf of agency goals and follow professionally developed procedures. There are variations in the amount of lay participation among agencies, depending on their stratagems for accomplishing their mission. Some emphasize community organization with local volunteers at the center of the action, particularly when fund raising is involved. Others that concentrate on expanding research and technology and evaluating medical interventions place lay participation in a more peripheral supporting role. The voluntary association has become, in effect, a quasi-official social resource in health, fixed firmly in the system, politically voluntary but structurally complementary to the official public health structure.

The voluntary health association continues to draw on the reservoir of Americans who are interested in and able to donate time in the interest of the community's welfare. A 1978 Gallup poll found that nearly 65 percent of those surveyed who lived in cities were willing (if given the opportunity) to work on solving local problems. Health-related activities accounted for about one-third of their interests. The Gallup study concluded: "Volunteerism is important not so much as a low-cost option for providing urban services (although there is a potential saving here), but as an effective way to improve the social fabric of our cities."[58] But it is clear that a substantial proportion of those who acknowledge their interest in volunteering have in mind an opportunity to provide a direct and concrete service in which the needs are visible and the benefits are immediate. This may be part of what appears to be widespread public disillusionment with governmental programs in the human services: a sense that national solutions to local problems have not worked or are not addressing current priorities and a belief that bureaucratic structures are not sufficiently accountable to the people. In part, then, we can speculate that there are factors in the recent political experience that push us toward the local, more directly accountable solutions to social problems. These push factors are complementary to psychosocial needs for individual identity, preservation of personal (or family or group) integrity, and the need to be needed.

Certainly the voluntary associations, hospitals, nursing homes, and the like continue to offer an avenue for lay involvement. But at the same time their limits of organization, roles, and goals, confined as they are to professional constructions of community health needs and priorities and bureaucratic constructions of procedures, do not necessarily respond to what the public now defines as involvement.

New patterns of volunteerism in health have proliferated in this period of political skepticism and alleged erosion of personal identity. They are part of a broad sweep of interest in options and alternatives to traditional definitions of the problem and orthodox forms of intervention. The search has been for ways of person-to-person help that minimize the limitations and liabilities of older forms of social response. Perhaps the best example of the new volunteerism in health are those helping activities in which a need is being met through the work of those who can identify with the need and can benefit most from the solution. The cocounseling relationship (peer service) is a case in point. As Bruce Baldwin and

Robert Wilson point out, the attractive features of this approach (as perceived by the client-providers) include informal style, accessibility with little administrative structure, present-oriented and practical help, anonymity, an egalitarian helping relationship, more felt acceptance of behavior and life-style, and fee-free service.[59] Clearly these attributes, relating specifically to peer counseling, cannot be applied uniformly to all forms of direct service volunteering. Expectations and qualifications of volunteers, styles of service, relationship with professional resources, and service goals vary widely among settings. Each volunteer modality contributes a perspective on the concept of direct service volunteering and raises pertinent questions of both benefits and limitations. Descriptive research on lay health service is hardly a decade old and has not yet related itself to a theoretical framework. It is an appropriate area for grounded theory research to elucidate and validate a theory of lay care-giving services based on the perceptions of those involved.[60] What are available now are mostly brief vignettes that describe a particular approach or program. The published literature is so meager that it is not possible to draw general conclusions or even to grasp the range of variation extant in lay voluntary services. The literature is useful, however, in contributing to an emerging catalogue of themes that highlight the rationale, process, structure, assets, and liabilities of this form of nonprofessional health care service.

We have chosen to amplify several of these themes as important to the general idea of lay voluntary service as a mediating structure in health. Our review focuses on the impetus for starting a lay volunteer service; recruitment and screening of volunteers; training the volunteer; the structure of volunteer programs; the economic value of lay volunteer service; and effects on volunteers and their clients.

### Impetus for Voluntary Lay Health Service

As noted earlier, forces in the current sociopolitical climate create a fertile environment for the growth of alternative health care approaches, particularly those where lay people at the local level can be personally involved in responding to neighborhood and community needs. What are the factors that appear to trigger lay volunteer programs in any given situation? Accounts of contemporary forms of lay volunteers in health service focus primarily on a *rationale* for the service rather than on questions of initial community interest and the initiating stimulus. Further, the intent of these reports is to show how a program operates and to evaluate its process and outcomes. The first generation of lay volunteerism in health associated with the youth counterculture movements of the 1960s has been succeeded by the initiatives of professional agencies, many of which were the earlier targets of young people in their quest for relevance, wholeness, and self-possessiveness.[61] Studies of lay volunteerism now begin at the point of agency interest with little or no acknowledgment of any prelude in the community's experience.

So we can say that the impetus for voluntary lay health service today, far from being an exclusively endogenous, free-standing, and spontaneous community response to the inadequacies of the professional care system, is encouraged by the professional resource itself as it attempts to modernize or even to survive. The Human Sexuality Information and Counseling Service of the University of North Carolina is illustrative.[62] It was apparent to the organizers of this service that increasing demand for sexual information and counseling could not be met within the framework of professional resources. The use of unpaid student volunteers was an acceptable and effective solution. Considered an alternative to professional services, the management of this peer-counseling program is nevertheless highly professional in its attention to training, quality control, and an emergent specialization of functions. The impetus for expanding coverage or adding new services can be expected to continue to come from the service system itself, responding to population needs and preferences as these are perceived by the volunteering staff and its professional advisers.

## Recruitment and Screening of Volunteers

Lay volunteers are becoming an integral component of such professionally organized outreach programs as crisis intervention centers and telephone hot lines. With this movement of volunteer activity into the mainstream of human services, the process of recruiting volunteers has moved from its earlier spontaneous form, when those interested merely stepped forward, to the present planned approach of inviting volunteer applicants and screening them. Indeed, the current practice of recruiting volunteers seems not to differ substantially from the way agencies go about recruiting professional workers. One could conclude, in fact, that the recruitment of volunteers applies a more conscious emphasis on affective qualifications, such as openness, warmth, involvement, and empathy, than would be true ordinarily in the selection of professional staff. These are the traits, after all, that were originally seen (and still remain) as compensatory for perceived shortcomings of professionals. In effect, the volunteer is selected both as an extension of professional services and as a mediating resource between the client and the system. The selection procedure can often be quite elaborate. For example, volunteers referred to the Suicide Prevention Center of Los Angeles were prescreened by the Los Angeles Mental Health Association and staff of the suicide center. Each applicant was then interviewed by at least three professional staff persons. All three interviewers had to be in agreement on acceptability. Finally, the candidates were given the Minnesota Multiphasic Personality Inventory (MMPI) and asked to write an autobiography.[63] Criteria for selection included maturity, responsibility, motivation, sensitivity, willingness to accept training and supervision, and ability to work in a group setting.[64] Interestingly, this selection process was specifically designed to discourage and eliminate volunteers who possessed many of the attributes of the earlier counterculture alternative mentality, in other words, to pose the problem within their own value system and to explore situations that may lie outside the limits of the established professional resource. Key professional staff of the Suicide Prevention Center of Los Angeles summarized their position:

> Certain volunteers were avoided. These were especially people looking for a way to gratify their own needs and to push their own individual conceptions of human problems and their solutions. Their investment was frequently in such areas as astrology, hypnotism, spiritualism, numerology, graphology and others. Often such persons were emotionally disturbed themselves, rigid, inflexible and tenuously organized. It was felt that such persons would not serve the agency, they would use it.[65]

Weeding out deviant personalities and deviant ideologies is one purpose (or result) of efforts to stabilize the role of volunteers in health care-giving agencies. A rather substantial literature has emerged on the predictive value of various tests (particularly the MMPI) in sorting out good from bad volunteers.[66] Reviewers of this transition from the open enrollment period for volunteers in the 1960s to the present screening process in closer proximity to professional values judge the situation as a positive and beneficial change. Gordon Holleb and Walter Abrams presented this view:

> It is our opinion that the present forms of these [alternative] programs represent an improvement over their initial stages. They are stable, effective, and accepted in their communities. They are providing a much more helpful service than the forerunner alternative programs. They are less ideologically radical and certainly less flashy than before, but they are more realistic and they seem built to last. They have, in sum, matured.[67]

The key is careful screening and acceptance of the governing ethic of the "employing" agency. In our review of the literature, it became apparent that screening is a key factor in accelerating the transition (or incorporation) of lay volunteers within established health agencies. As this device increases in sophistication and wider application, it is safe to predict that fewer accepted volunteers will be separated, divorced, or widowed, have only a high school education, drink heavily, experience depression, ever consider suicide or attempt it, ever have been treated by a psychologist or psychiatrist, or be young (around twenty-three years).[68] Increasingly, the volunteer will more resemble the professional provider (or at least the provider's concept of self) than the clients. This clearly represents a compromise with an earlier tenet of volunteerism, that the social distance between helper and client be minimal as a basis for easy communication and credibility.

It is altogether possible that published reports on the selection of volunteers are biased in favor of programs in more orthodox health settings, such as crisis centers, community mental health centers, and cancer outreach programs. Volunteerism as a modality of service in other settings, particularly educational settings, may not have undergone such a dramatic break with its earlier form. Peer counseling, for example, by definition, adheres to the "social similars" model and, because it operates in an environment that emphasizes education, development, and growth rather than diagnosis, treatment, and cure, may retain a higher level of tolerance for deviance among and between volunteers and clients.

Recruitment and screening of volunteers, it has been shown, can attract and accept a highly diverse group without sacrificing integrity or compromising the protection of clients from incompetents. One program reports on how the selection *process* itself can act to encourage self-deselection. Beatrix Hamburg and Barbara Varenhorst described an approach to self-selection in a high school cocounseling program that is compatible with the earlier values of volunteerism while achieving both system *and* client acceptability:

> The training program was set up in such a way that initially, and at various points during the course of training, hurdles and obstacles were designed to weed out students of lesser commitment. Students had to initiate action to get in, find their own transportation to the training meetings, attend meetings on their own time, check a designated mailbox for important notices, call if they could not attend a meeting, and make up missed sessions. Requirements of this kind provided behavioral evidence of a degree of responsibility and commitment that was necessary. . . .
>
> Finally, the program was based on the theory of self-selection and volunteer participation. No student was denied admittance if it was requested. No pretraining screening took place . . .[69]

Clearly, this model offers no guarantee against ineptitude, but it allows for the test of competence to be actual behavior rather than a priori judgment. Once again, an educational setting may be unusually conducive to using a system of self-selection through overcoming built-in hurdles in the process of becoming a qualified volunteer. On the other hand, the self-selection strategy has been used routinely in staffing crisis intervention centers and seems effective in yielding highly motivated volunteers while maintaining an egalitarian approach to open recruiting.[70]

### Training the Volunteer

Two propositions govern the training of lay volunteers in health service, regardless of the complexity of the tasks they are ultimately to perform: (1) the volunteers' natural resources of maturity, sensitivity, motivation, and caring are the key attributes required, and (2) the most effective training is practical experience. It is the goal of training programs to preserve and enhance the inherent skills of the volunteer in a way that is both credible and efficient. The aim is not to mimic professionals, but to make a natural and creative resource available in service to the community.

To achieve this ideal requires a balanced strategy that in essence assesses the starting competence of the volunteer, provides opportunities for reenforcing it, and adds additional skills that complement the style of the volunteer. Whereas the earliest forms of volunteer training have been criticized as "haphazard and informal,"[71] one may now in some instances see the pendulum swing toward excessive control and professionalization. Most probably, the bulk of volunteer training falls somewhere between these extremes, but the trend seems unequivocally in the direction of using lay volunteers in more substitutionary roles (in contrast to the earlier roles of adding a new service). This leads to increased emphasis on training in professional skills and styles, modified (simplified, condensed) for use by the lay volunteer.[72] Furthermore, as lay volunteerism has grown as a significant service resource, it has began to cross the boundaries of professional function. And there is no doubt that lay volunteerism has also raised concerns among friends of the movement that the time has come to establish and enforce performance standards, including screening and training, that would help protect gains already made and legitimate the volunteers' role as a stable component of the health and social service resource. Attempts to set standards for suicide prevention centers are well documented. Jerome Motto concludes a review of standard-setting efforts with the caution that:

> In the future development of suicide prevention and crisis services, standards can play an important role, not only as a stabilizing influence but as a divisive force as well. . . . If . . . leaders in the field insist on a significant and rapid departure from the direction of the past decade, a severe strain will be put on those who are in the mainstream of this work.[73]

There are portents of power struggles for control of the volunteer service modality.

From the limited pool of published accounts and surveys of lay volunteer programs, one gets the impression that training remains heavily an on-the-job learning experience sandwiched between didactic lectures. Some of the more commonly reported learning themes are clinical and social aspects of the problem at issue, diagnostic methods, concepts of communication, counseling skills, and the use of community resources. Educational methods that seemed to be favored are lectures, role playing, case histories, tape-recorded interviews, observation of professionals at work, and work under supervision. The variations on content and methods appear rather modest, the greatest variation occurring in the length of training, the amount of supervision, and the extent of continuing education. There is a clear reliance on older volunteers to socialize newcomers into the ways of the system.

Standards for training are being promulgated and probably will most immediately affect programs of national scope (suicide prevention, rape counseling centers); yet there appears to remain a commitment to keep the training within bounds of cost and time. Parsimony in the training process can be accomplished without sacrificing quality of lay volunteer performance. Robert Carkhuff and Charles Truax review the evaluative research on minimally trained volunteers, which corroborates their own study of a short-term didactic-experiential training of lay group counselors. These authors conclude "that a specific but relatively brief training program, devoid of specific training in psychopathology, personality dynamics, or psychotherapy theory, can produce relatively effective lay mental health counselors.[74]

### Structure of Volunteer Programs

From the volunteer hot lines of the late 1950s and early 1960s to the present centers for crisis intervention, there has been a tendency for more face-to-face contact between client and volunteer, more emphasis on counseling, follow-up, and quality control. As a consequence, more structure is required to achieve a broader set of goals and to maintain services as a reliable and continuous community resource with strong ties to professional services.

Professionals increasingly appear as initiators of lay voluntary services, and to various degrees they design (or guide) the structure of the service. As one national survey of suicide prevention and crisis programs found, most of the programs by 1968 "were originally stimulated or implemented by concerned clergy who, in almost all cases, quickly involved psychiatrists and other mental health professionals in consultant or advisory capacities.[75] The church appears to offer a particularly sensitive setting in responding both to the needs of congregants and to the use of congregants as health volunteers in matters involving mental health support. It develops naturally out of the pastoral counseling experience. A contemporary example is crisis counseling for members of the gay community. Michael Enright and Bruce Parsons described the design of a gay counseling program in Salt Lake City, which began from one church's recognition of a growing demand for meeting the needs of the gay community effectively, efficiently, and equitably.[76]

Of course, the use of lay volunteers as substitutes for or extensions of professional roles in established health service programs results in highly structured management designs to which the volunteer is subjected. Indeed, some lay volunteer roles are so highly structured and controlled that the only remaining attribute that distinguishes them from professional staff is their payless status.

Regardless of the extremes of lay volunteer service with regard to management design, one can find some minimal structural elements of the service programs that protect client, volunteer, and agency. Aside from training, which in some form is universal, all programs involving lay volunteers appear to keep records and to have some system to protect the anonymity (or at least privacy) of the clients. Record keeping has become an essential part of the crisis services, like hot lines, as these services seek to improve follow-up and referral to various professional resources. But along with this bureaucratic necessity came a commitment to maintain what was perhaps the central value of the earlier forms of lay volunteer action: to protect the client's identity. It was not just a matter of protection, but also to encourage (or at least symbolize) a nonjudgmental service provided by people one could trust as brothers or sisters. As Baizerman observed, "The social value and social norm of anonymity were functional for relating themes of the Counterculture and the Movement with specific social expectations of behavior and with hotlines."[77]

Evaluation now appears an almost universal aspect of lay volunteer structure, regardless of its level of independence as a community service. Considered an innovation in service delivery, lay volunteers in established agency programs have been scrutinized often at a level that matches or may even exceed measurements of the effectiveness of counterpart health professionals. But it is clear that evaluative criteria are the product of professional and agency perspectives and values. In effect, there is a prescription that volunteer services are qualitatively similar to counterpart professional roles. Thus the yield of volunteer care is measured in terms that mask whatever might be the unique effects of volunteer care or place them in a lower order of priority. A long-range effect might be an erosion of the morale of volunteers given that their reasons for volunteering and their expectations of client benefits may not be rewarded. One observer anticipated that this, together with other structural impositions on volunteer service, could result in volunteerism's "going full circle and finding small volunteer services starting to emerge anew."[78] At present, evaluation strategies appear most concerned with legitimating the volunteer's role as a basis for reshaping agency policy. In reality the process may result simply in normalizing alternative services as a resource for service expansion rather than service revision.

### Volunteer-Professional Relations

It should come as no surprise that as lay volunteers become more closely affiliated with established agencies or become more established themselves, their contribution is sometimes greeted with ambivalence by health professionals who function as supervisors or consultants. There is, of course, the immediate issue of work boundaries and the almost inevitable desire for more responsibility once volunteers feel comfortable with their role and begin to see additional possibilities for service. Just as professionals seek advancement, so do volunteers respond to a need for new challenges and new opportunities to capitalize on their experience. How and where can workers go, should they legitimately aspire to tasks of more complexity and responsibility? The answer to this question derives from the intricate chemistry of the program's genesis (lay or professional), the level of professionalism of the professional staff, the power level (self-confidence) of the volunteer, the parity of volunteer-professional training (common elements), and the nature of the volunteer's role in agency decision making. And overarching all of this are the more general aspects of the professional-volunteer relationship, particularly shared ideology and mutual respect.

Reports on the lay volunteer experience do not usually reveal these important elements of the work situation. An exception is a study of ten crisis centers reported by Robert McGee.[79] Volunteer respondents were asked to relate what characteristics of professionals in their opinion identified them as "helpful and valuable" to the program and also what characteristics made them "undesirable and unacceptable" to the volunteer. Volunteers characterized positively those professionals "who demonstrated an acceptance of the volunteer as a capable person" and "who did not appear threatened or defensive about letting volunteer workers assume major responsibility." There was a clear recoiling from professionals who were patronizing or who dominated decision making. Interestingly, volunteers were most positive toward professionals who were "willing to learn from the volunteer." And, of course, perceived competence, dedication, and energy were characteristics the volunteers valued highly in their evaluation of professionals. In fact, it is striking that criteria applied by volunteers are not at all different from the attributes of volunteers that are highly regarded by professionals. The difference lies in the power to apply such criteria in program development and operations. Professionals may use them in selecting, training, and supervising volunteers. Volunteers, on the other hand, have no such opportunity with reference to professionals. The implications of this imbalance in opportunities mutually to determine compatibility in the volunteer-professional relationship are likely to be most obvious in agency-based volunteer programs in contrast to volunteer-peer enterprises, as in the earlier versions of hot lines. When volunteers are seen as employees, unanimity of goals and mutuality of effort, which are central in the value of volunteerism, are bound to be compromised. How this affects clients, volunteers, and professionals needs considerable study beyond presently available anecdotal material. This matter has not been of as much concern as the selection of volunteers. A good amount of internal restructuring may be necessary to achieve the kind of mutual respect required to optimize the benefits of a professional-volunteer system of service. Mechanisms for volunteer inputs in the selection, monitoring, and evaluation of professionals would seem to be an appropriate way of preventing discordance and promoting a constructive and creative relationship.

Socialization of the agency-based volunteer into the values and procedures of the agency is, of course, key to the role relationships involved in the service. Volunteers who cannot (will not) accept supervision, for example, are systematically screened out of agency-based programs, thereby eliminating those who are potentially high risk as a source of conflict. Is it not possible that those rejected on this criterion might well be persons whose initiative and resourcefulness (as reflected in their independence) are more in concert with the unique values of volunteerism than is true of their accepted counterparts?

## Economic Value of Lay Volunteer Services

Information on the cost of lay volunteer service is scarce and, with few exceptions, inadequate for comparison purposes. First, there are the usual difficulties associated with budget analyses, such as definition of the accounting unit, definition of cost itself (to whom), in-kind contributions unaccounted for (donated space), regional variations, and difficulties in time comparisons, to name a few. Further, the concept of budget may not be appropriate for voluntary activities that function on a money-available basis and are not able to develop a budget projection. These limitations are almost uniformly applicable to the earlier modes of lay health volunteerism. With the ascendancy of lay volunteers as an integral component of established service agencies, we can expect (and already see) the earmarking of funds for volunteers and implementing of accountability procedures. If for no other reason, agencies (as part of the plan to make secure volunteer resources) must document their belief that "utilizing paraprofessional volunteers was much less costly to an agency that was experiencing vanishing funding sources."[80]

For hot lines and similar services that are not performed face to face, the identification of direct costs and budgeting are easily determined. It is another matter for personal contact services in which space, supporting resources, professional time sharing, and a multitude of indirect costs must be accounted for.[81] The cost implications of volunteer turnover also are a factor for all programs, particularly those where selection and training investments are substantial. One point is clear: volunteer programs are not free of cost. Savings accrued in salary costs must be increasingly discounted as the volunteer service moves into the overall service mix of an agency. At this time there are few satisfactory analyses of such volunteer costs, much less an estimate of cost-benefit or cost-effectiveness. A reasonable concern here is to achieve a notion of cost-benefit-effectiveness that incorporates those items as aspects of volunteer, client, and agency. This is especially relevant in the cost measurement of a human service design in which the benefits to providers may be as important as the benefits to consumers. The mutual aid benefits inherent in the role of the lay volunteer cannot be ignored.[82]

## Effects on Volunteers and Clients

Lay volunteers of the counterculture era in America represented a powerful example of helper and client solidarity in values, credibility, and nonpunitive support. The structure of this support was nonhierarchical, and its functions were cast in a social rather than in a clinical model. Under such conditions, volunteer service was obvious in its contribution of empathic understanding and its social and political acceptability and accessibility.[83] As noted, volunteer services have undergone considerable mutation as they have become incorporated in agency-based services. Yet, despite a situation of regulatory impositions in the form of professional selection, training, and supervision, lay volunteers appear to have retained a substantial part of their special, perhaps unique, relationship to clients; and when they are forced to conform too rigidly to a professional model, they have been known to rebel or withdraw. It seems safe to conclude that lay volunteers, whether they serve in face-to-face, continuous support roles or through telephone one-time encounter hot lines, are at least able to demonstrate trace elements of the earlier pure volunteer character of their role.[84]

But it is not only the potential loss (or retention) of the positive benefits of volunteer help that is relevant to the present status of volunteer-client relations. There is also substantial commentary on nonproductive and often counterproductive aspects of lay volunteerism. Those are most dramatic and visible among volunteers working in palpably stressful situations. Volunteers as cancer patient counselors are perhaps the most vivid example. Mark Kleiman, Joanne Mantell, and Esther Alexander reported on the experience of cancer patients as volunteers in assisting other cancer patients and their families.[85] The evaluators of this demonstration identified multiple negative effects on both volunteer and client. Those include (for the volunteer) exhibiting covert resentment toward dying patients, overidentifying with patients, reflecting guilt and depression, urging their own values on patients, and managing the lives of patients. With regard to effects on clients, there were instances where patient families were subject to volunteers' attempts to increase their guilt in order to motivate the families to be more supportive. But even with these serious negative contributions, the cancer patient demonstration was judged as positive overall: "Volunteers frequently built rapport by focusing initial interactions on their common experiences with cancer. This eased the tasks of both patients and volunteers in making the transition to the pressing issue of death."[86]

It is clear, however, that the benefits to the volunteer may equal those to the client. Most reports of volunteer programs give special attention to this point. Many of the immediate benefits are related to personal growth, greater awareness of human behavior, and sensitivity to the needs of others. Increased respect for the integrity of individuals is also evident as volunteers shake off initial illusions of themselves as saviors. Learning to respond to clients and to empathize without taking over is another important outcome for volunteers. And, of course, volunteering provides through training and the conditions of supervised experience a rich curriculum of ideas and skills in communicating, listening, counseling, interpreting feedback, learning about available community resources, and making (and following through on) referrals. For some, the volunteer experience may serve as a stimulus to seek academic preparation and qualifications as professional workers. In at least one setting (a suicide prevention center), this latter outcome was consciously encouraged even though the process of professionalizing the volunteer may have sacrificed essential values of the volunteer role:

> As the volunteers have grown in experience and skills, they have developed as mental health counselors. . . . In our Center [their identity with the profes-

sional mental health field] was constantly encouraged by attitude and precept so that volunteers readily adopted the professional stance. . . . Perhaps as a direct result, three persons have returned to school with a professional goal in view.[87]

In attempting to gain a realistic perspective on the benefits of lay volunteer programs for clients, we are faced with a literature that tends to report on programs on the whole judged successful. They are reasonably balanced in their reports of weakness and strengths, but objective surveys of volunteer efforts and their impact on clients remain rather sparse and limited in venue. But if we accept these limitations and view published evidence with suitable caution, it is not unreasonable to conclude that, under a wide range of circumstances, lay volunteers do make substantial contributions to clients and, even more broadly, to the community as a humane environment.[88]

There is no doubt that evaluation of lay health volunteer programs, both free standing (volunteer controlled) and agency based, is spotty and perhaps even inappropriate. Lack of funds and of access to valid observations, the limits of descriptive research (no controls), the constraints imposed by the requirement of anonymity, are all complicit in making evaluation and a global judgment difficult. Methods have been proposed to build evaluation into volunteer programs,[89] but the very nature of volunteerism as an endogenous social movement with highly variable goals and conditions of operation make the appeal most practical for the larger, agency-based volunteer programs, which have established networks.

We can only comment on the groundswell of public interest in getting involved and the powerful continuing attraction of lay volunteerism in health. The balance of benefits and liabilities remains problematic, but we are inclined to believe that at the very least the volunteer movement caused the reexamination of its social potential in health care as more than a passing fad of limited appeal and limited application.

The lay volunteer service in health meets the criteria of a mediating structure. To what degree and in what ways this resource is being eroded or compromised as a functioning mediating force is of great concern, particularly as it operates in the more established program settings.[90] Our view is that lay volunteerism will continue to regenerate around new social and health needs of society, regain its pure role status as it defines a new problem and raises social consciousness, and then become professionalized and institutional-ized as a regular component of established services. This should not be construed as a pessimistic or cynical view. We should, on the contrary, look at the process as a natural source of institutional change, a powerful contribution to the humanization of professional services. The requirement for mediation in health care is constantly shifting. It is testimony to the efficacy of lay volunteerism that it responds sensitively to priorities and emergent needs and casts the original die of a new perspective on meeting those needs.

## A CLOSER LOOK: RAPE CRISIS CENTERS

Let us now examine a specific type of volunteer organization that also has some of the characteristics of a mutual aid group, the rape crisis center. The rape crisis center is a powerful example of a lay organization formed in response to a regrettably common community problem, the crime of rape and what was perceived to be unsatisfactory treatment of the rape victim by hospitals, police, and the courts. These centers can take many forms, and their functions and structure may differ somewhat from one com-munity to the next. But rape occurs in small towns as well as large ones, in suburbs as well as in cities, and it happens to women of all ages, classes, and races. Groups have organized all across the country to respond to the problem in remarkably similar ways. Awareness of the problem of rape has grown tremendously in the last decade, with the dissemination of several highly publicized books and the convening of national conferences. And these have undoubtedly spurred further organization locally. The remarkable increase in the number of these centers around the country cannot be seen as the successful carrying out of anyone's master plan. Their spontaneous generation can be attributed to the pervasive influence of the women's movement during the late 1960s and early 1970s with its focus on the rights of women to control their own bodies.

We will look at the forms these centers have taken, the functions they most commonly perform, the women who make them up, and the impact they are having on local institutions, their communities, and, in some cases, even the law. Finally, we will look at the way one rape crisis center in New York City was organized and how it has developed into a program that seems to benefit everyone concerned.

Though of course rape crisis centers are involved in the legal and criminal justice aspects of rape, their focus has always been on the often neglected victims of the crime, and underlying all their activities is a concern for these victims' mental and physical health. Thus, like other mediating structures, rape crisis centers are multifunctional and differ a great deal from one another in their emphasis on the medical, psychological, and legal aspects of rape.[b] Since the one thing that unites all rape crisis centers is a primary concern for the well-being of present and potential victims of rape, the social support functions are common to them all.

### Historical Development

There are many different types of rape crisis centers, started by different groups with different reasons for being concerned about victims of rape. Though many have been feminist in their political orientation, not all have been so, as the authors of the only national study of such centers point out.[91] Besides feminist collectives, volunteer or service organizations, church groups, civic organizations, ad hoc committees, professional associations, social clubs, and more traditional women's organizations have undertaken rape-related projects, some of which have resulted in the provision of some form of service for rape victims. For the purpose of this chapter, all these groups will be considered mediating structures if they depend on volunteers for the provision of services.

But if other groups have subsequently become involved, credit for the initial raising of this issue to its present level of social awareness must certainly go to the women's movement. The establishment of rape crisis centers is one manifestation of the concern the current women's movement has had, from its inception, for health issues and for the control women have and do not have over their own bodies. In fact, the women's health movement has emerged as a strong and growing force in the critique of the way medical services are provided to all people in this society and has contributed to the

---

b. Our emphasis in this section is on the social support functions of these centers, not their medical-legal or court-watching functions, though of course these are important.

clarification of the alternatives.[92] Not all the activities of the women's health movement are as sensational as the concern with rape; most of their efforts are directed toward the far more mundane and universal concerns of routine health maintenance and care. Two observers of the women's health movement trace its origins to the popular health movement of the nineteenth century.

In this century the focus of the women's movement on health and body issues probably began with the political action to change abortion laws. Through the medium of feminist consciousness-raising groups, concern spread to sexuality, contraception, medical, especially gynecological, practice, and mental health. A movement periodical estimated in 1974 that there were 1,200 such health-oriented feminist groups in the United States.[93] The enormously popular *Our Bodies, Ourselves* was first published in 1971 and has been a best seller ever since.[94] The first feminist health clinic was also established in 1971 in Los Angeles. Since then many others have been opened; they offer gynecological care and occasionally abortions, prenatal care, and counseling.[95] Many of these clinics have incorporated their critique of traditional medical services into a program of self-help and health education that makes care givers and care receivers mutual participants in the process. The literature of the women's health movement has also attacked certain specific medical practices, such as the use of the hormone DES, now known to cause cancer; the performance of unnecessarily radical mastectomies; and overmedication during childbirth.

The issue of rape also has been raised by the women's movement from its beginning. The development of rape crisis centers and the criticism of the current medical and legal treatment of the rape victim should be seen as occurring simultaneously with these other developments. Both feminist and nonfeminist writers agree that the origins of rape crisis centers are in the women's movement and that without it they would never have arisen. The first raising of the issue took place in 1971, with the publication of an article in *Ramparts*,[96] and with the New York Radical Feminists Speak-Out on Rape.[97] The resulting discussions, many of which took place in consciousness-raising groups, led to several forms of collective action, the most important of which were the rape crisis centers. The first centers were started in 1971, in Washington, D.C., New York, Michigan, and California, though none of these groups were aware of the others at the time. Other groups in other cities soon followed, as these first groups began to publicize their efforts.[98] It is interesting to see the increase in the number of such centers listed in recently published studies of rape. From thirty-one centers listed in one 1974 book,[99] to 136 centers in thirty-eight states and the District of Columbia identified in a study by the Center for Women Policy Studies,[100] the numbers appear to be large and growing. In 1977 there were also twenty-two rape crisis centers in Canada.[101]

After an initial period of self-education, many of these groups took as their first task an investigation of the treatment of rape victims in their own community, by their own police, hospitals, and courts. In most cases it was found that victims were often handled insensitively and ineptly and their cases pursued unsuccessfully. They found that only a small proportion of cases were reported to the police and that the apprehension, trial, and conviction of a rapist is relatively rare. There was considerable criticism of hospitals, too, for the way rape victims were frequently treated in the emergency room. Women who had been raped complained about waiting for hours before being seen, because their physical injuries seemed minor. They often had to wait in public areas of emergency rooms where they were loudly identified as "a rape." Some hospitals and doctors even refused to examine rape victims to avoid having to become involved in a legal action. Other hospitals had inadequate procedures for collecting evidence or allowed inexperienced interns or residents to perform the examination. Often the evidence that was collected did not stand up in court. Even worse, however, was the insensitivity displayed to rape victims, whose mental and emotional state was unquestionably vulnerable. Snide remarks by emergency room personnel were frequently reported, as were unsolicited opinions by the examining doctor as to whether or not the woman was "really" raped. To make matters worse, women who had received this inadequate treatment were often billed large amounts of money. As one study put it, "Women all over the country have been trying to understand what hospitals have against rape victims.[102] A study undertaken by the federal Law Enforcement Assistance Administration has gone so far as to liken the visit to the hospital as a second rape: "She was raped in private during the crime; she has now been raped in public."[103]

The hospital emerged as a prime target of criticism for several reasons, not just humanitarian ones. Besides adding insult to insult and injury, hospitals were frequently lax in starting and maintaining the "chain of evidence," so that cases brought to trial were lost. Thus there was a significant motivation on the part of law enforcement agencies and district attorney's offices, in addition to feminist and community groups, to revamp hospital procedures. Though it may be said that rape crisis centers are more concerned with the victim's welfare and that law enforcement is more concerned with the improved collection of evidence, these goals are certainly not in conflict. Rape victims who are treated well are far more likely to cooperate in the prosecution of their case, and the successful conviction of the rapist is nearly everyone's ultimate goal.

### Functions of Rape Crisis Centers

Given these diverse motivations and the uniqueness of community values and problems, it is not surprising that rape crisis centers work out their responses to the problem of rape in different ways. Writing in 1974, one author saw three types of "rape groups" emerging. The first she called the "clearinghouse groups": large and well-known groups who have acquired a national reputation and who concentrate on publicity, education, and the publication of materials for use by other rape groups. The second type she called the "multiple center." These groups also serve educational purposes but are in addition involved in direct services to rape victims, usually by means of a twenty-four hour hot line that provides legal, medical, and police referrals and peer counseling. They may also sponsor mutual aid groups for women who have been raped and educational programs for police, district attorney, and hospital staffs. The third type of group identified was the "expertise group." These groups tended to specialize in one area, such as court watching or counseling. The author observed that most groups went through an initial period of about a year of meetings, research, and negotiations before actually deciding on the focus their group would take.[104]

In what follows, we will be looking at the functions of groups that fall into the second and third categories, those that work directly with rape victims. It is in its work with rape victims that a rape crisis is a mediating structure in the fullest sense. The rape crisis center, in the person of a counselor/advocate,[c] acts as a mediator between the rape victim and numerous institutions, the police, the hospital, and the courts. These victim-related services represent the inner face of the mediating structure in relieving human suffering through one-to-one interaction. Later we will look at the outer face, which has acted to bring about some important political and legal changes.

The rape crisis center plays a mediating role that is in some ways supplemental to the natural support networks rape victims have, but it may also act to mobilize those resources in support of the victim. In one study of ninety-two rape victims at Boston City Hospital, it was found that the great majority of the women, seventy-three, were able to turn to some social network for support.[105] This was most often their family, even if they lived in another city. The crime of rape, however, can have almost as strong an impact on the husbands, friends, and families of victims as it does on the victims themselves. Feelings of guilt, fear, and anger at the situation can sometimes get in the way of the support the victim needs. One group of men in Philadelphia has started a rape counseling service for the husbands, boyfriends, or fathers of rape victims, because it found that these men often needed an outlet for the expression of these negative feelings.[106] The rape crisis counselor/advocate has resources of knowledge and experience in dealing with what is almost certainly a new and shocking situation for rape victims and their families. And for some victims who do not have other sources of social support or who are unwilling to call on them, the counselor/advocate may provide all their emotional support.

The knowledge that the counselor/advocate has to offer the rape victim may be divided into three areas, which we will look at: the legal, medical, and psychological aspects of rape.

One of the first things that research into the problem of rape in our society discloses is that the conviction rate of men accused of rape is very low. When it is taken into account that in only a small proportion of cases are arrests made and men brought to trial on

c. The term "counselor/advocate" will be used throughout to designate the volunteers, because it clearly conveys the roles they play vis-à-vis rape victims on the one hand and medical and legal institutions on the other.

charges of rape, this number seems even smaller. One study of the way police in Canada classified reports of rape as "founded" or "unfounded" revealed some of the ways in which complex social influences affect these ostensibly objective legal processes.[107] In addition, the fact that so few women report the crime—authorities generally agree that reported rapes account for only 5 to 10 percent of all rapes committed—makes a conviction for rape rare indeed.[108]

The role of rape crisis centers is relevant to both of these problems. The counselor/advocate can perform a paralegal function by giving the rape victim the information she needs to decide whether to report the rape to the police or not. The counselor/advocate can tell the woman what to expect in the police investigation and the medical examination for collection of evidence. If the initial encounter takes place over the telephone, the counselor/advocate can advise the rape victim about which hospital to go to and may offer to meet her there and accompany her through the process. Some rape crisis centers may continue their contact with the rape victim as her case proceeds through the criminal justice system and act as her advocate in dealing with the district attorney. The counselor/advocate can help the rape victim make decisions that are in her own best interests by discussing all her alternatives with her and letting her know what to expect. Some women who might not have reported the crime to the police may be persuaded to go through with it because they know they will not be there alone. Others may decide, through their discussion with the counselor/advocate, that to report the crime would be too painful or that the chances of obtaining a conviction would be too small to warrant the action. In either case, the victim will be making an informed decision.

One of the most important effects of rape crisis centers has been the development and adoption by hospitals of strict protocols for the examination of rape victims and the collection of evidence. The medical treatment of rape victims is basically: treatment for any injuries she may have received in the assault, the collection of evidence, and treatment to prevent venereal disease and pregnancy. The examination is not performed to determine whether or not rape occurred; that is a legal, not a medical, question. The medical examination can only determine evidence of recent intercourse. Although standardized procedures for the medical treatment of rape victims have been available since 1970[109] and do not in themselves necessitate the presence of a rape crisis counselor/advocate, few hospitals put them into practice until an organized group pressed for their adoption.

The role of the counselor/advocate with regard to the medical examination is primarily informational, but in some hospitals she may be permitted to provide emotional support through her presence in the examining room. Counselor/advocates can discuss all aspects of the examination with the rape victim beforehand, including the pelvic examination, which may be new and quite distressing to some women. The counselor/advocate can also discuss the prophylactic treatment for venereal disease, which in most cases is given as a matter of course. The possibility that the rape victim may become pregnant as a consequence of the rape should also be raised. If there is a likelihood of pregnancy, some hospitals administer DES, but this should never be done without first advising the woman of possible hazards of the drug and making her aware of other alternatives so that she can make her own decision. In sum, the role of the counselor/advocate is not a medical one: she performs no examination and provides no treatment. But she can counsel the victim so that she knows what to expect, and in some hospitals she may even act as her advocate in dealing with the emergency room staff.[110]

The counselor/advocate can play her most important role, however, in meeting the psychological needs of the rape victim. A woman who has been raped has been through a humiliating and degrading experience. Although her body has been violated, her wounds may be more psychological than physical, making her inordinately sensitive to the way she is treated by those around her. On the other hand, the rape victim should not be made to feel that her reactions are symptoms of mental illness and that she needs psychiatric help. This is one of the primary values of peer counseling. Counselor/advocates recognize that the normal reactions to the crime of rape can be quite varied and at times extremely intense, reflecting individual styles of coping. Rape crisis centers recognize that peer counseling is most appropriate in dealing with initial reactions to the crime and providing immediate temporary support. A continuing inability on the part of a rape victim to return to a state of normal functioning may indicate the need for professional help, and the counselor/advocate can then make an appropriate referral. Brodyaga's national study of rape crisis centers showed that none of the programs attempted to provide intensive or long-term therapy for rape victims.[111]

The majority of women who are raped are not mentally ill and do not become so as a result of the rape. The presence of peer instead of professional supports during the initial phases of reaction and adjustment conveys to the rape victim the expectation that she will probably be able to deal with this situation without experiencing lasting emotional trauma.

There is a substantial body of literature developing on the subject of the psychological reactions of rape victims, most of it facilitated by rape crisis centers. The most important finding overall has been that the normal reaction to rape can take many forms of expression and that rape victims should be encouraged to use the method of coping they find most comfortable. One early study focused on two main emotional styles, which the authors called "expressed" and "controlled."[112] About half the women they interviewed were moderately verbal or quite talkative, and they welcomed the opportunity to talk with the counselor about their experience. The other women were more guarded and quiet, tending to keep their feelings to themselves. The authors conclude that there are no right or wrong ways to respond to a rape and that the most important service a counselor can provide is emotional support, expressed by not leaving the woman alone and by listening carefully to what she has to say.

The later research of these authors examined the responses of women who had been raped, immediately after the incident and during a follow-up period of up to one year.[113] They discovered a pattern of reactions to rape they called the "rape trauma syndrome." They found that women who had been raped usually experienced an acute phase of disorganization immediately after the crime, which generally lasted about two to three weeks. During this period women frequently experienced physical trauma and emotional reactions expressed as fear, humiliation, anger and, self-blame. For most women, however, this period was not long-lived, and most moved readily into the second phase of the syndrome, characterized by a process of reorganization. Efforts to cope with their new situation included changing places of residence, changing telephone numbers, and taking trips, often to visit families. The authors mentioned ego strength and social network support as important factors affecting their ability to cope.

Other research has emphasized the need of rape victims to regain feelings of control over their immediate surroundings. The radical helplessness and vulnerability they experienced during the attack can, unfortunately, often be reinforced by either insensitive or infantilizing treatment by the police or hospital staff. The counselor/ advocate is trained to be aware of this danger and to facilitate the reassertion of control by encouraging the woman to make immediate decisions regarding her care and treatment. The rape victim needs to feel involved from the very start in the prosecution of her case and in the prevention or treatment of pregnancy and venereal disease, rather than feeling herself to be the passive object of procedures she may not understand or is not ready for.[114]

As mentioned earlier, rape crisis centers do not try to fill needs for long-term psychotherapy other than providing referrals to appropriate professional resources. Some groups, however, have sponsored mutual aid groups for rape victims who may want some continuing nonprofessional support.[115]

### Structural Forms

Most rape crisis centers begin as nonhierarchical collectives, in which each woman is involved in all aspects of decision making. An early survey of feminist rape crisis centers revealed that all the groups valued their nonauthoritarian structure. They also tended to be quite small, made up of three to fifteen members.[116] Though this style of organization may be ideologically attractive, there are problems of lack of efficiency, leading to overwork and subsequent "burnout." Hence many groups have evolved a somewhat more structured approach in the form of task forces or steering committees, which attempt to delegate responsibility for the sake of efficiency while preserving each individual's sense of responsibility to the group as a whole.[117]

The most common service provided by rape crisis centers is the twenty-four-hour telephone hot line. This is often the first service provided by such groups because it is relatively easy to set up and to publicize. It shares the characteristics of peer counseling hot lines described earlier. Often the last four digits of the number are 7273, which spells RAPE, making the number easier to remember. The hot line can serve as an emergency number for women who need help immediately, as a source of referrals and information, or as a source of support for women who may have been raped some time previously and just want to talk with someone. The anonymity of the hot line may be especially important to women who are afraid to tell anyone else or who are unsure whether to report it to the police. Staffing a twenty-four-hour hot line from a central office requires an immense amount of volunteer time, and it may be impossible for a small group to handle. Some groups have found solutions to this problem by hiring an answering service or using a tape recorder when no one is on the line. An improvement over these systems is the telephone-switching service available with pushbutton phones, which allows the hot line number to ring in the on-duty counselor/advocate's home.[118]

In the national survey of rape crisis centers, about 80 percent of the centers reported attempts to establish a relationship of cooperation with the police, hospitals, and prosecutors so that a counselor/advocate could accompany a rape victim in all her contacts with these agencies. About half of that 80 percent reported fair to poor relationships with local hospitals in their attempts to institute changes in emergency room procedures for treating rape victims, including allowing counselor/advocates to be present.[119] Working with and trying to change the practices of complex bureaucratic institutions such as hospitals is considerably more difficult than establishing a new, small-scale institution and fraught with far more political difficulties. As one feminist struggling with these issues of compromise put it:

> Their [Brodyaga et al.'s] suggestions assume the necessity for cooperation, e.g. the patient advocate, they state, should have a good relationship with the hospital. But then, how can she advocate? On the other hand if she doesn't have a good working relationship how effective will her advocacy be?[120]

But affiliation or cooperation with an institution can greatly increase the number of women helped; so such attempts at cooperation will probably continue. One rape crisis center in Philadelphia is located in a hospital, and it was able to assist 800 rape victims in its first year.[121]

Counselor/advocates can be of significant help to both rape victims and emergency room personnel if they are allowed to play a significant role in caring for the rape victim at the hospital. Nursing journals have lately given some attention to the nursing care of rape victims in the emergency room, counseling sensitivity, patience, and a willingness to listen.[122] The reality of the situation in the hospital, however, is often less than conducive to the kind of patient listening suggested. Busy nurses in understaffed emergency rooms may feel frustrated that they cannot give the time they would like to the rape victim, whose wounds may be invisible. In addition, there is the ever-present danger of professional burnout for those who become emotionally involved in these crisis situations on a day-to-day basis.[123]

Counselor/advocates, on the other hand, have no reason for being in the emergency room except on behalf of the rape victim and thus have no conflicting demands on their time or energy. Besides performing the roles of explaining treatment procedures and providing emotional support, the counselor/advocate can be of great practical help. She may make telephone calls, get coffee or cigarettes, or talk to the rape victim's relatives or friends if she is asked to do so. Some hospitals have a storage place for nonmedical supplies that rape victims frequently need: underwear and clothing to replace that which is taken as evidence, douches for use after evidence is collected, mouthwash, and petty cash for food or carfare. The counselor/advocate's freedom to pursue these roles depends to a large extent on hospital policies and the cooperation of emergency room personnel. Jurisdictional disputes may indeed arise, but they are not impossible to overcome, as will be shown. Furthermore, the benefits of an effective counselor/advocate role can accrue to everyone concerned, not least the volunteers themselves.

## The Volunteer Counselor/Advocate

According to the national survey of rape crisis centers, most volunteers are young middle-class white women between the ages of twenty and forty who are college educated or students.[124] Often these groups were started in the first place because the women had known each other through feminist organizations or consciousness-raising groups.

Only about half the groups identified themselves as feminist organizations, however. Only a small percentage of the volunteers were themselves victims of rape. This finding was shared by another survey, which found that few members of rape crisis centers had been raped, but that some groups were founded by women who knew someone who had been raped and then badly mistreated by the police or the hospital.[125]

Thus, despite these groups being formed on the basis of shared values, they should be clearly distinguished from mutual aid groups in that interaction is not always based on shared experience. And unlike members of mutual aid groups, who are trained by their experience, the volunteer counselor/advocate has to learn both techniques and information before she can be very helpful to a rape victim. Training in these groups is similar to that in other volunteer organizations offering peer counseling services. Training is usually conducted by more experienced volunteers, who may be aided by medical or legal professionals. To be genuinely helpful to rape victims, counselor/advocates need to be fully informed about all aspects of rape and all of the local community's ways of dealing with the problem. Training is usually conducted in several sessions before a prospective volunteer is permitted to go on call. Some groups may extend the training through monthly meetings where members can discuss problem cases and get feedback and support from each other.

But training cannot produce the willingness and motivation necessary for what can be a physically and emotionally exhausting job. One study of the volunteers at a rape crisis center in Charleston, South Carolina, showed considerable psychological maturity on the part of the volunteers.[126] A group of counselor/advocates were given a battery of psychological tests, which showed them to be significantly less neurotic than national norms.

Because it is a volunteer service, the rape crisis center can provide types and amounts of service that would be prohibitively expensive to provide professionally. For example, staffing a twenty-four-hour phone line requires more than three times the amount of labor in a full-time workweek. And even in the biggest city hospital, there are many shifts during which no rape victims come in for treatment, which would leave a specialized professional with nothing to do. In a sense, the things volunteer counselor/advocates do—getting up in the middle of the night to sit with a stranger in an emergency room or answering a phone all night long—are things that only dedication could motivate.

The problem of professional burnout has been mentioned, but the possibility of volunteer burnout should also be raised. Small groups in which a few women attempt to be on call continuously will probably not last very long. Ideally, the group should have enough members so that each volunteer has time to rest and regroup between what may be emotionally draining experiences. The group should also have institutionalized ways in which it can function as a support system for itself.

### The Rape Crisis Center and the Larger Community

Like other mediating structures, the rape crisis center also has an outer face directed to changing the social and political situation in which rape occurs. Once established, most rape crisis centers find they are frequently asked to speak to local community groups, schools, hospitals, block associations, and church groups. Such meetings serve the purposes both of informing the public about the help available for rape victims and possibly of preventing some crimes through education. One group listed the topics usually covered in their talks: the myths and facts about rape, the injustice of existing rape laws requiring corroboration and evidence of resistance, self-protection, and what to do and expect if someone is raped.[127] Some groups may also undertake public education on a larger scale through television and the print media. A number of groups have published their own pamphlets on how to start a rape crisis center or on rape prevention and self-defense.[128]

Rape crisis centers are also playing a leading role in research on the crime of rape, the reactions of victims, and the way the crime is handled by other institutional structures. They are in a unique position to conduct research on rape because of their intimate contact with the victims. Often they have access to information that could be gotten through no other channel. For instance, women who have not reported the crime to the police and may not even have told their families may feel safe calling a hot line, because they know their anonymity is protected.

The subject of confidentiality is an extremely important one if a rape crisis center is to function responsibly. It also illustrates very well the conflicts that can arise when a center attempts to serve institutional objectives other than the immediate, self-perceived needs of the rape victim. Such issues can become especially complex when the center depends on funding from an institutional source, such as a district attorney's office, whose goals may not always exactly coincide with the rape victim's welfare.

The issue of funding is of serious concern to all rape crisis centers. Even if they are staffed completely by volunteers, there are expenses for telephones, office supplies, printing, and rent. Many rape crisis centers are located in spaces donated to them in private homes, YWCAs, women's centers, churches, colleges, or community organizations. But many groups have become "victims of their own success."[129] As public interest and awareness have grown, their services have become more and more in demand. Many centers found that they needed some full-time staff members to keep up with the demand for public speaking, answering mail, and keeping records. Some writers have advised groups to incorporate as nonprofit organizations and to establish themselves as tax exempt so as to attract tax-deductible contributions and foundation funding.[130] But attracting and keeping funding means keeping records and writing applications and reports, and those activities take talent and time away from providing services. When combined with the problems of compromise and cooptation that may occur when a rape crisis center affiliates with another institution, the resulting tensions can sometimes break groups apart.[131] One suggestion that has been made to solve these problems has been for federal funding to go directly to rape crisis centers. Making money available would decrease the need for centers to spend so much of their time in fund raising, and having the money go directly to the center would reduce the control other institutions have over them.[132]

Rape crisis centers have found that, to aid rape victims, changes had to be made in the ways institutions handled the crime after the fact. This is a big enough job in itself, but most groups soon realized that other, deeper structural changes were also imperative. One of the reasons for very low conviction rates, besides the lack of adequate techniques for collecting evidence, has been the existence of state laws that require the testimony of a witness other than the victim, make admissible into evidence the rape victim's past sexual history, and mandate high sentences, including life imprisonment, for rape. The effect of these laws has been an unwillingness by prosecutors to bring rape cases to trial, an unwillingness of rape victims to have their past sexual relationships publicly scrutinized, and an unwillingness of juries to convict because the punishment may seem excessively severe. Centers have actively undertaken to change these laws in the states of New York, California, Michigan, Iowa, and Florida, among others, with some success.[133]

The long-term goal of social changes undertaken by rape crisis centers, however, is to eliminate the need for themselves. The open expression of such a goal is unique to volunteer organizations that have nothing to gain from maintaining the status quo.[134] Changing the law and providing protection and support for the victims can go a long way toward encouraging more women to report the crime and making it easier for prosecutors and juries to convict the guilty. And through a combination of education for potential victims and deterrence for potential rapists, rape crisis centers hope to prevent some of these crimes in the first place.

The following account of one volunteer rape crisis center illustrates many of the processes and issues raised in this chapter, including the burnout and professionalization of volunteers, the benefits of a nonprofessional approach to crisis intervention, and the volunteer organization's potential for bringing social change to institutions and communities.

### The Rape Intervention Program at St. Luke's

The Rape Intervention Program in the emergency room of St. Luke's Hospital on the Upper West Side of Manhattan began operating in 1977. It is a volunteer program with a paid half-time coordinator who is herself a volunteer, sixty volunteer advocates from the neighboring community, and supervision from the hospital's departments of psychiatry and obstetrics-gynecology.

The program was initiated by several members of a women's health collective, a feminist psychiatrist on the staff of the hospital, and a medical student, who met with representatives of the hospital's emergency room and social services staffs. Through review of the hospital records, it was discovered that approximately ten to fifteen rape victims were being treated in the emergency room each month, and there was a strong consensus that the hospital and the community had a responsibility to do something for these women.

A proposal was made to the hospital, and potential volunteers were recruited through advertisements in the local student and community newspapers. They were screened and trained by the steering committee, made up of equal numbers of volunteer advocates and hospital staff. Volunteer advocates are usually on duty one night per month and are called immediately by the triage nurse when a rape victim comes into the emergency room.[135] They live in the neighborhood of the hospital, and arrive there within fifteen minutes. The volunteer advocate talks with the rape victim before any treatment is undertaken, unless the victim has injuries that require immediate attention. Only after the advocate has had a chance to explain the procedures and their purpose and secured the woman's permission to proceed is the gynecologist called. The advocate usually remains in the examining room with the rape victim, if she gives her permission, reviews the treatment plan the doctor has prescribed, and answers questions. The advocate also informs the woman about the importance of follow-up treatment. There is a follow-up medical visit with a nurse practitioner.

Since the program began, it has served more than 305 victims of sexual assault, who have ranged in age from two to eighty-three. The largest number of rape victims have been between the ages of eighteen and forty. About 50 percent have been black, about 34 percent white, and 16 percent Hispanic and other, roughly reflecting the population of the community.

One of the most important goals of the program has been to minimize psychological trauma through immediate intervention. By restoring the rape victim's sense that she is cared for and that she has some control over her surroundings, the advocate can go a long way toward reducing feelings of helplessness and vulnerability. The experience of the St. Luke's Hospital program has been that only a small percentage of all rape victims required immediate psychiatric consultation, and in these cases the psychiatric problem usually antedated the rape.[136] There are three kinds of psychological follow-up: The advocate calls the rape victim the next day to find out how she is doing and reminds her of the availability of the hospital's social work staff. The psychiatric social worker follows the victim and her family during the crisis period and after and provides the continuity and expertise to supplement the advocate's role. A third, relatively new aspect of the program has been group therapy for adult rape victims. Two self-help groups have been started for women who had first been seen in the emergency room. These groups became very cohesive and supportive for their members, especially those whose cases came to trial.

Currently, there are sixty volunteer advocates in the program. The majority are young white women, with a small minority of Oriental, Hispanic, black, and older women. There are graduate students, medical students, teachers, ministers, and others. According to the codirector of the program, the volunteers have been completely reliable in being near their telephones when they are on duty and in responding promptly.[137] There are three Spanish-speaking volunteers, who are available at any time. The program has experienced about a 50 percent turnover of volunteers each fall when a new training session has been held, but some of the volunteers who were trained in the first group are still involved in the program. This continuity has led to greater awareness of the needs of volunteers who take on such emotionally demanding and highly responsible tasks, which may lead to their "burning out" as volunteers. A group of volunteers is meeting regularly to discuss their feelings about their experiences. Some of the issues that have come up are fears for their own personal safety, knowing what they do about crime in their own neighborhood; overidentification with some of their clients; and strains on their personal relationships, especially with husbands and roomates, who at times have had to bear the brunt of their strong emotional reactions. The other noticeable effect on a group of volunteers who are becoming extremely knowledgeable about the treatment of rape victims is that they want more responsibility. The response of the hospital staff has been a positive recognition of their expertise and respect for their judgment.

The program has received funding from outside the hospital to pay part-time salaries of the coordinator of the program, who is responsible for scheduling, conducting meetings, and running the program on a day-to-day basis, and a social worker who has organized the group therapy sessions for rape victims. Other expenses have been for supplies, materials, including a videotape project, and research and evaluation, which has produced several published articles and an annotated bibliography. The grants have been given by a private foundation and a bank.

In general, the program has been very well received by the hospital staff and administration. "They still don't understand how we can work with a steering committee and be so democratic," commented a member of the steering committee, "it's not the way they're used to operating." The emergency room nurses, who were often too busy to give such time-consuming care to rape victims, are especially pleased. And the program's growing reputation in the community is certainly good for the hospital as a whole. Several articles about the Rape Intervention Program have appeared in local community newspapers. They have more requests for speakers, from schools, banks, colleges, and community groups, than they can handle.

The program inspires a great deal of pride in those who are associated with it. The volunteers have the satisfaction both of helping other women on a one-to-one level and of having a significant impact on a major community institution. As the coordinator put it, "What we're doing is so concrete. That's what makes it exciting. We're changing consciousness in the hospital and outside the hospital, and changing structures as well."

## IN RETROSPECT

Mediating structures are social resources that contribute to individual growth and adaptation. They are a source of strength, identity, and protection. They perform life-satisfying functions, which are so taken for granted that their existence often becomes known only through their loss. Damage to mediating structures, as we have noted, is revealed in the rise in morbidity, both personal and social. The inherent benefits of mediating structures are difficult to substitute or compensate for. Public programs for nurturance and for building and maintaining identity often perpetrate the very hazards they are designed to prevent. Homes for the elderly and centers for senior citizens are examples of the limits of social institutions planned to compensate for insufficiencies of the mediating resource. Social welfare programs generally, professional medical care, and public education are all to some extent compensatory for mediating structures. Some are necessary and desirable in the complex modern world, but all are compensatory. The industrial development of these social agencies has tended to obscure their compensatory status, creating an illusion of their total effect as primary, central, and dominant. It is no surprise, then, to see massive efforts to expand, improve, and broaden access to these agencies. Social research has focused on the character of their function and social policy on their manipulation in the public interest. In contrast, research and policy interest in the health, welfare, and educational contributions of mediating structures has been modest. The Western world has come to view some of these functions as almost exclusively professional, institutional, or governmental. Health care is a powerful case in point. We have defined the cause of ill health in terms of the professional health care system, and we have limited its solution to the absence or presence, to the quality and efficiency, of that system. Only recently have the steep rise in the costs of such services and awareness of the limits and liabilities of professional care raised interest in alternatives. Individual, family, and community nonprofessional resources in health are being rediscovered. As we assemble documentation of nonprofessional health resources, particularly the contributions of individuals and families, a picture of the health care "system" emerges that is dominated by the *lay* resource. Indeed, in the mix of lay and professional health resources, the professional sector is obviously supplementary, although the specific effect each has on the other is unclear.

The professional construction of the health world today is cast primarily in industrial and bureaucratic terms. As an industry, economic modeling of demand is accounted for in the use of purchasable goods and services. As a bureaucracy, the health system is measured in terms of occupations and the organization of work. The cost, distribution, and benefit of the product are all determined within the values of the industry. Even in the measurement of social effects, the choice of indicators of health status reflects professional definitions of deviance. The industrial-bureaucratic world of medicine is to nonprofessional health care as an aquarium is to the sea. It possesses an ecosystem, an integration of its elements. But its management and control are external to its functioning parts. The rules of governance, of growth and innovation, are imposed by a definition of the health resource that is restricted to components of the health marketplace. This eliminates the nonmarket health care provided by individuals, families, and the informal, nonprofessional helping network. The aquarium of the professionally constructed health world is neither a simulation of the sea of health activity nor a true complement of it. The professional model of health care is not linked either in policy or in practice to the condition, changes, or exigencies of health care in the nonprofessional sector. Indeed, the professional care system is largely unaffected by the usual roles of supply and demand. Further, organized professional services by and large stand as *disjecta membra* from shifts in patterns of disease, increasing lay competence in personal health, and changes in public tastes and preferences in health care.

There are many reasons why we must reorient our thinking about the health care resource, but the most obvious reason is that of truth, a value that transcends objectivity. Research on professional care has yielded a plethora of objective data, but these data fall short of the full reality of health care and as a result contribute a biased perspective, a misrepresentation of both the function and the contribution of professional care in society. In effect, a powerful myth emerges, which forecloses, or at least forestalls, critiques of assumptions about the role of professional care, its limits, benefits, and liabilities. It constitutes the doctrinal basis for the promulgation of professional resources, the charter for the serviced society, which provides a service for every need and, where there is no need, creates a need for every service.[138] The results are visible in the increasing medicalization of social problems and processes to meet the maintenance and growth needs of the health industry, now the third largest employment sector in the United States, with nearly 5 million employees. Add to this the nonproductive and counterproductive implications of this "growth industry," and one can sense the economic and political difficulties faced in challenging the view that professional health care is synonymous with the total health care resource. The surprise of lay persons when confronted with information that the vast proportion of *all* health care is self-provided is some indication of how firmly the professional care concept is established. An adjustment of the public perspective on health care is an essential condition for reformulating the definition both of what constitutes the "crisis" in health and of what constitutes the full range of solutions.

Our concern in this book has been to create the basis for reconsideration, and in some cases reconciliation, of mediating structures in health and professional resources. Our full attention to the nonprofessional domain should not be construed as a detraction or even distraction from the essential contribution of professional care. The precise points we are making are that strengthening the lay sector in health is the most reasonable and generous way of making more efficacious the role of professional care. The second and corollary point is to consider an approach to professional care development that in its own interests is sensitive to the benefits of partnership with the lay health resource.

Our examination drew on critiques of the professional health resource stemming directly from the experience of mediating structures. Most of these critiques are defensive in that they argue not so much for the reduction of medical care, although that is sometimes sought, but for preservation of its essential benefits and protection from its erosive effects. Criticisms of professional health care within this framework are raised as residual aspects of the central theme and only when they pertain to procedures, programs, or policies that hinder, weaken, or threaten the effectiveness of the social resource in health.

The argument for a reappraisal of the health care resource to include the social resource of mediating structures is profoundly conservationist: to conserve and nurture the health care functions of individuals, the family, the neighborhood, and the community.

## REFERENCES

1.  P.H.J.H. Gosden, *Self-Help: Voluntary Associations in the Nineteenth Century* (London: B.T. Batsford, 1973), p. 4.
2.  Alfred H. Katz and Eugene I. Bender, "Self-Help Groups in Western Society: History and Prospects," *Journal of Applied Behavioral Science* 12 (1976): 265-82.
3.  Gosden, *Self-Help*, p. 22.
4.  Richard H. Shryock, "Sylvester Graham and the Popular Health Movement," *Mississippi Valley Historical Review* 38 (1931): 172-83.
5.  William B. Walker, "The Health Reform Movement in the United States, 1830-1870" (Ph.D. diss., Johns Hopkins University, 1955), p. 113.
6.  Regina Markell Morantz, "Nineteenth Century Health Reform and

Women: A Program of Self-Help," in Guenter Risse, Ronald Numbers, and Judith Leavitt, eds., *Medicine without Doctors* (New York: Science History Publications, 1977), pp. 73–94.

7.  Shryock, "Sylvester Graham," pp. 179-82.

8.  William G. Rothstein, *American Physicians in the Nineteenth Century* (Baltimore: Johns Hopkins University Press, 1972), p. 159.

9.  David J. Rothman, *The Birth of the Asylum* (Boston: Little, Brown, 1971).

10. Sheila Rothman, *Woman's Proper Place: A History of Changing Ideals and Practices, 1870 to the Present,* (New York: Basic Books, 1978).

11. Ibid., pp. 124–27.

12. Richard Carter, *The Gentle Legions* (Garden City, N.Y.: Doubleday, 1961), chap. 3.

13. Ibid., chap. 4.

14. Eliot Freidson, *Patients' Views of Medical Practice* (New York: Russell Sage Foundation, 1961), p. 146.

15. Marvin B. Sussman, "The Isolated Nuclear Family: Fact or Fiction," *Social Problems* 6 (1959): 333–40.

16. Ibid., p. 335.

17. Jeffrey Colman Salloway, "Medical Care Utilization among Urban Gypsies," *Urban Anthropology* 2, no. 1 (1973): 113-26.

18. Allan Horwitz, "Family, Kin, and Friend Networks in Psychiatric Help-Seeking," *Social Science and Medicine* 12A (1978): 297-304.

19. Karen Kay Petersen, "Kin Network Research: A Plea for Comparability," *Journal of Marriage and the Family* (May 1969): 271-80.

20. Irving K. Zola, "Healthism and Disabling Medicalization," in Ivan Illich et al., *Disabling Professions* (London: Marion Boyars 1977), pp. 41-67.

21. See, for example, John B. McKinlay, "Social Networks, Lay Consultation and Help-Seeking Behavior," *Social Forces* 51 (March 1973): 275-92.

22. Irving K. Zola, "The Concept of Trouble and Sources of Medical Assistance, to Whom One Can Turn, with What and Why," *Social Science and Medicine* 6 (1972): 673-79.

23. Sydney H. Croog, Alberta Lipson, and Sol Levine, "Help Patterns in Severe Illness: The Roles of Kin Network, Non-Family Resources, and Institutions," *Journal of Marriage and the Family* 34 (February 1972): 32-41.

24. Ibid., p. 40.

25. Berton H. Kaplan, John C. Cassel, and Susan Gore, "Social Support and Health," *Medical Care* 15, no. 5, Supplement (May 1977): 47-58.

26. Harvard PSRO, "Information and Consumer Choice: The Case for Public Disclosure of Health Services Data" (February 1975).

27. Lisa F. Berkman and S. Leonard Syme. "Social Networks, Host Resis-

tance, and Mortality: A Nine-Year Follow-Up Study of Alameda County Residents," *American Journal of Epidemiology* 109 (1979): 202-3.

28.    Alfred H. Katz, "A Discussion of Self-Help Groups: Haven in a Professionalized World?" (Prepared for Mediating Structures Project Conference on Professionalization, American Enterprise Institute, New York City, May 11-12, 1979).

29.    Ibid, p. 10.

30.    Ibid, p. 10-11.

31.    Alan Gartner and Frank Riessman, "Self-Help Models and Consumer Intensive Health Practice," *American Journal of Public Health* 66, no. 8 (August 1976): 784.

32.    George S. Tracy and Zachary Gussow, "Self-Help Health Groups: A Grass-Roots Response to a Need for Services," *Journal of Applied Behavioral Science* 12, no. 3 (1976), special issue: *Self-Help Groups,* pp. 381-82.

33.    Sol Tax, "Self-Help Groups: Thoughts on Public Policy," *Journal of Applied Behavioral Science* 12, no. 3 (1976), special issue: *Self-Help Groups,* p. 448.

34.    Thomas J. Powell, "The Use of Self-Help Groups as Supportive Reference Communities," *American Journal of Orthopsychiatry* 45, no. 5 (October 1975): 756-64.

35.    Lowell S. Levin, "Self-Care and Health Planning," *Social Policy* 8, no. 3 (November-December, 1977); 47-54, Eugene C. Durman, "The Role of Self-Help in Service Provision," *Journal of Applied Behavioral Science* 12, no. 3 (1976), special issue: *Self-Help Groups,* pp. 433-43.

36.    Alfred H. Katz and Eugene I. Bender, eds., *The Strength in Us: Self-Help Groups in the Modern World* (New York: New Viewpoints, 1976), p. 36; Alfred Katz, personal communication, June 4, 1980.

37.    Alan Gartner and Frank Riessman, *Self-Help in the Human Services* (San Francisco: Jossey-Bass, 1977).

38.    Ibid., pp. 159-76.

39.    Durman, "Role of Self-Help," p. 442.

40.    Kurt W. Bock and Rebecca C. Taylor, "Self-Help Groups: Tool or Symbol?" *Journal of Applied Behavioral Science* 12, no. 3 (1976), special issue: *Self-Help Groups,* p. 307.

41.    Ivan Illich et al., *Disabling Professions* (London: Marion Boyars, 1977).

42.    Bock and Taylor, "Self-Help Groups,", p. 296.

43.    Stephen F. Jencks, "Problems in Participating Health Care," *Self-Help and Health: A Report* (New Human Services Institute, Queens College, City University of New York, September 1976), p. 95.

44.    Robert H. Moser, *Diseases of Medical Progress: A Study of Iatrogenic Disease* (Springfield, Ill.: Charles C. Thomas, 1969).

45.  Alfred Katz's comments, reported in the minutes of the opening plenary session of a conference "Self-Help and Health" (New York, June 8, 1976) and published in *Self-Help and Health: A Report* (New Human Services Institute, Queens College, CUNY, New York, September 1976), p. 11.

46.  Helen I. Marieskind and Barbara Ehrenreich, "Toward Socialist Medicine: The Women's Health Movement," *Social Policy* 6, no. 2 (September/ October 1975): 40.

47.  Eugene I. Bender and Alfred H. Katz, "Self-Help as a Social Movement" (paper presented at the Pacific Sociological Association Annual Meeting, Scottsdale, Arizona, May 3, 1973), mimeo., p. 5.

48.  Alfred H. Katz and Eugene I. Bender, "Self-Help Groups in Western Society," *Journal of Applied Behavioral Science* 12, no. 3 (1976), special issue: *Self-Help Groups*, p. 281.

49.  Gartner and Riessman, "Self-Help Models," p. 784.

50.  Katz, "A Discussion of Self-Help Groups," p. 11.

51.  Ibid.

52.  James S. Gordon, "Special Study on Alternative Mental Health Services," *Task Panel Reports Submitted to the President's Commission on Mental Health,* Vol II, (Washington, D.C.: 1978), pp. 376–410.

53.  Ibid., pp. 379–81.

54.  Morton A. Lieberman and Leonard D. Borman, "Self-Help and Social Research," *Journal of Applied Behavioral Science* 12, no. 3 (1976): 455–56.

55.  First International Conference on Self-Help and Mutual Aid in Contemporary Society, Dubrovnik, Yugoslavia, September 10–15, 1976.

56.  Richard Carter, *The Gentle Legions* (Garden City, N.Y.: Doubleday, 1961).

57.  Paul E. White, Lowell Levin, and Sol Levine, "Community Health Organizations and Resources," in Howard E. Freeman and Sol Levine, eds., *Handbook of Medical Sociology,* 3rd ed. (Englewood Cliffs, N.J.: Prentice-Hall, 1979), pp. 347–68.

58.  George Gallup, "The Cities: Unsolved Problems and Unused Talents," *Antioch Review* (Spring 1979).

59.  Bruce A. Baldwin and Robert R. Wilson, "A Campus Peer Counseling Program in Human Sexuality," *Journal of the American College Health Association* 22 (June 1974): 403.

60.  Barney Glaser, *Theoretical Sensitivity: Advances in the Methodology of Grounded Theory* (Sociology Press, 1978).

61.  Michael Baizerman, "Toward Analysis of the Relations among the Youth Counterculture, Telephone Hotlines, and Anonymity," *Journal of Youth and Adolescence* 3, no. 4 (1974): 293–06.

62.  Baldwin and Wilson, "A Campus Peer Counseling Program," pp. 399–404.

63.  Sam M. Heilig et al., "The Role of Non-professional Volunteers in a Suicide Prevention Center," *Community Mental Health Journal* 4, no. 4 (1968): 288.

64.  Ibid., p. 289.

65.  Ibid.

66.  David R. Evans, "Use of the MMPI to Predict Effective Hotline Workers," *Journal of Clinical Psychology* 33, no. 4 (October 1977): 1113–15.

67.  Gordon B. Holleb and Walter H. Abrams, *Alternatives in Community Mental Health* (Boston: Beacon Press, 1975), p. 7.

68.  Lawrence S. Schoenfeld, John Preston, and Russel I. Adams, "Selection of Volunteers for Telephone Crisis Intervention Centers," *Psychological Reports* 39 (1976): 725–26.

69.  Beatrix A. Hamburg and Barbara B. Varenhorst, "Peer Counseling in the Secondary Schools: A Community Mental Health Project for Youth," *American Journal of Orthopsychiatry* 42, no. 4 (July 1972): 570.

70.  Robert K. McGee, *Crisis Intervention in the Community* (Baltimore: University Park Press, 1974), p. 214.

71.  Holleb and Abrams, *Alternatives in Community Mental Health*, p. 28.

72.  See the example of Heilig et al., "Role of Non-professional Volunteers."

73.  Jerome A. Motto, "On Standards for Suicide Prevention and Crisis Centers," *Life-Threatening Behavior* 3, no. 4 (Winter 1973): 256.

74.  Robert R. Carkhuff and Charles B. Truax, "Lay Mental Health Counseling: The Effects of Lay Group Counseling," *Journal of Counseling Psychology* 29, no. 5 (1965): 430.

75.  Anson Haughton, "Suicide Prevention Programs in the United States—An Overview," *Bulletin of Suicidology* (July 1968): 25.

76.  Michael F. Enright and Bruce V. Parsons, "Training Crisis Intervention Specialists and Peer Group Counselors as Therapeutic Agents in the Gay Community," *Community Mental Health Journal* 12, no. 4 (1976): 383–91.

77.  Baizerman, "Toward Analysis," p. 301.

78.  Motto, "On Standards for Suicide Prevention," p. 257.

79.  McGee, *Crisis Intervention in the Community*, pp. 106–7.

80.  Enright and Parsons, "Training Crisis Intervention Specialists," p. 385.

81.  Eleanor E. Bauwens and Linda H. Belt, "The Value of Volunteers in Family Planning Clinics," *Family Planning Perspectives* 9, no. 4 (July/August 1977): 169–72.

82.  Connie Stuetzer, Diane Fochtman, and Jerome L. Schulman, "Mothers as Volunteers in an Oncology Clinic," *Journal of Pediatrics* 89, no. 5: 847–48.

83.  Heilig et al., "Role of Non-professional Volunteers," p. 289.

84. James E. Carothers and Lorene J. Inslee, "Level of Empathic Understanding Offered by Volunteer Telephone Services," *Journal of Counseling Psychology* 21, no. 4 (1974): 274–76.

85. Mark Allen Kleiman, Joanne E. Mantell, and Esther S. Alexander, "Rx for Social Death: The Cancer Patient as Counselor," *Community Mental Health Journal* 13, no. 2 (1977): 115–24.

86. Ibid., p. 123.

87. Heilig et al., "Role of Non-professional Volunteers," p. 294.

88. Robert J. Gregory, "The Rap House and Volunteers: Helpful or Harmful?" *British Journal of Addiction* 73 (1978): 103–6; Michael F. Enright and Bruce V. Parsons, "Training Crisis Intervention Specialists"; Robert Carkhuff and Charles B. Truax, "Lay Mental Health Counseling"; Christopher Bagley, "An Evaluation of Suicide Prevention Agencies," *Life-Threatening Behavior* 1, no. 4 (Winter 1971): 245–59.

89. David Lester, "The Evaluation of Telephone Counseling Services," in David Lester and Gene W. Brockopp, eds., *Crisis Intervention and Counseling by Telephone,* (Springfield, Ill.: Charles C. Thomas, 1973), pp. 276–86.

90. John M. O'Donnel and Kathi George, "The Use of Volunteers in a Community Mental Health Center Emergency and Reception Service: A Comparative Study of Professional and Lay Telephone Counseling," *Community Mental Health Journal* 13, no. 1: pp. 3–12.

91. Lisa Brodyaga et al., *Rape and Its Victims: A Report for Citizens, Health Facilities, and Criminal Justice Agencies* (Washington, D.C.: National Institute of Law and Criminal Justice, 1975).

92. Marieskind and Ehrenreich, "Toward Socialist Medicine," pp. 34–42.

93. Women's Health Forum, "Women's Health Movement: Where Are We Now?" *Health Right* 1 (1974).

94. Boston Women's Health Book Collective, *Our Bodies, Ourselves,* 2d ed. (New York: Simon and Schuster, 1976).

95. Marieskind and Ehrenreich, "Toward Socialist Medicine," p. 39.

96. Susan Griffin, "Rape: The All-American Crime," *Ramparts* 10 (1971): 3.

97. Noreen Connell and Casandra Wilson, *Rape: The First Sourcebook for Women* (New York: New American Library, 1974).

98. "How to Start A Rape Crisis Center" (Washington, D.C.: Rape Crisis Center, 1972).

99. Andra Medea and Kathleen Thompson, *Against Rape* (New York: Farrar, Straus, and Giroux, 1974), pp. 148–49.

100. Brodyaga et al., *Rape and Its Victims,* pp. 327–34.

101. Lorene Clark and Debra Lewis, *Rape: The Price of Coercive Sexuality* (Toronto: Women's Press, 1977), p. 191.

102. Connell and Wilson, *Rape,* p. 198. All the previously mentioned works also contain references to inadequate hospital treatment.

103. Brodyaga et al., *Rape and Its Victims.*
104. Connell and Wilson, *Rape,* pp. 191–92.
105. Ann Burgess and Lynda Holmstrom, "Rape Trauma Syndrome," *American Journal of Psychiatry* 131 (1974): 981–86.
106. Carol V. Horos, *Rape: The Private Crime, a Social Horror* (New Canaan, Conn.: Tobey, 1974), p. 97.
107. Clark and Lewis, *Rape.*
108. Susan Brownmiller, *Against Our Will: Men, Women and Rape* (New York: Simon and Schuster, 1975), p. 175.
109. American College of Obstetrics and Gynecologists, *ACOG Technical Bulletin* No. 14 (July 1970). Reprinted in Connell and Wilson, *Rape,* pp. 203–6.
110. Good summaries of the medical needs of the rape victim are available in Connell and Wilson, *Rape,* pp. 207–13; and Brodyaga et al., *Rape and Its Victims,* sect. 2.
111. Brodyaga et al., *Rape and Its Victims,* p. 133.
112. Ann Burgess and Lynda Holmstrom, "The Rape Victim in the Emergency Ward," *American Journal of Nursing* 73 (1973): 1740–45.
113. Burgess and Holmstrom, "Rape Trauma Syndrome."
114. Brodyaga et al., *Rape and Its Victims,* p. 124.
115. Clark and Lewis, *Rape,* p. 192.
116. Connell and Wilson, *Rape,* p. 185.
117. Brodyaga et al., *Rape and Its Victims,* p. 124.
118. Ibid., pp. 132–33.
119. Ibid., p. 135.
120. Pauline Bart, "On Rape," *Women's Health* 1 (1976): 21–22.
121. Brodyaga et al., *Rape and Its Victims,* pp. 136–37.
122. Darlene Sredl, Catherine Klenke, and Mario Rojkind, "Offering the Rape Victim Real Help," *Nursing '79* (July 1979): 38–43; Burgess and Holmstrom, "Rape Victim in the Emergency Ward."
123. Eleanor Schuker, "Psychodynamics and Treatment of Sexual Assault Victims," *Journal of the American Academy of Psychoanalysis* 7 (1979): 553–73.
124. Brodyaga et al., *Rape and Its Victims,* p. 126.
125. Connell and Wilson, *Rape* p. 182.
126. Connie L. Best and Dean G. Kirkpatrick, "Psychological Profiles of Rape Crisis Counselors," *Psychological Reports* 40 (1977): 1127–34.
127. Connell and Wilson, *Rape,* pp. 239–40.
128. Brodyaga et al., *Rape and Its Victims,* p. 129.
129. Brodyaga et al., *Rape and Its Victims,* p. 125.
130. Horos, *Rape,* p. 114.
131. Connell and Wilson, *Rape,* p. 187.

132.  Connell and Wilson, *Rape,* chap. 4.

133.  Details of specific changes can be found in Brodyaga et al., *Rape and Its Victims,* App. IV-A.

134.  Connell and Wilson, *Rape,* pp. 156, 178; Clark and Lewis, *Rape,* p. 191.

135.  For one volunteer advocate's account of what it means to be on call in this program, see Sarah Darter, "A Ministry to Rape Victims," *American Baptist* (March 1979).

136.  Eleanor Schuker, "A Treatment Program for Rape Victims," *Alaska Medicine* 20 (1978): 48-55; Schuker, "Psychodynamics and Treatment of Sexual Assault Victims," p. 563.

137.  Ibid. p. 53.

138.  John McKnight, "Professionalized Service and Disabling Help," in Ivan Illich, ed., *Disabling Professions* (London: Marion Boyars, 1977), pp. 69-91.

# 5 MEDIATING STRUCTURES AND HEALTH POLICY

Many aspects of mediating structures are far from being entirely clear. The tools available to improve clarity may not be impartial given their origins in sciences and professions with their own vested interests. Moreover, the conceptual simplicity of mediating structures and their expression in common experience make it difficult to establish their special integrity in health care.

Those limits and concerns color discussion of the implications of mediating structures for health policy. We are surrounded by health resources that are profound in their ordinariness. They are often (usually) recognizable only through purposeful study, raised to consciousness as it were, for a given purpose at a given time and measured against given criteria. Unlike the definitions and perceptions of physicians or nursing homes, those of nonprofessional, informal health resources follow no standard classification scheme. Mediating structures are culturally determined, highly variable in form and function, and often obscured by their primary identification as family, church, or friend. Policy formed in response to such health resources cannot be expected to rely on traditional methods of calculating costs or benefits or negotiating trade-offs among competing political interests. Health policy traditionally deals with the known competence, productivity, and jurisdiction of professional resources. This is a finite system of resources predictable, accountable, and in some measure controllable by the system itself. One knows what to expect when more hospital beds are added, more doctors are trained as family practitioners, or a national health service corps is deployed. There is a reasonable basis for predicting, and therefore planning, the impact of new technology and increased efficiency in emergency medical services. Where allocation and deployment are feasible strategies, planning is an appropriate management tool. On the other hand, when policies take mediating structures into account, planning must be more reactive than assertive, more protective than promotive. The flow of policy should be from the mediating resource toward the professional resource and designed to supplement and reinforce. Policy must follow a strategy of maximizing the service potential of each successive component of the health care system, starting with the informal lay resource and identifying residual functions for increasingly larger and more complex social resources. Nearly fifty years ago, this perspective on planning social policy was put forward by Pope Pius XI as the "concept of subsidiarity":

> It is a fundamental principle of social philosophy that one should not withdraw from individuals and commit to the community what they can accomplish by their own enterprise and industry. So, too, it is an injustice and at the same time a grave evil and a disturbance of right order to transfer to the larger and higher collectivity functions which can be performed and provided by the lesser and subordinate bodies. Inasmuch as every social activity should, by its very nature, prove a help to the members of the body social, it should never destroy or absorb them.[1]

## ASPECTS OF MEDIATING STRUCTURES OF SPECIAL RELEVANCE TO HEALTH POLICY

The notion of subsidiarity forms the philosophic nexus between the lay and professional components of the health care system. Its validity as a guiding perspective is anchored in certain beliefs about the reality, utility, and unity of both lay and professional resources. Beliefs about the lay resource, buttressed with what evidence is available, have been expressed throughout this book, but it may be helpful to summarize them here as a basis for our view of the implications of mediating structures for health policy. We shall set forth those aspects of mediating structures we believe are most important for policy makers to take into account when developing laws and rules.

## A Broader Definition of Health Care

It is no longer accurate (it never was realistic) to define health care strictly in terms of professional resources. Like data on the professional resource, our knowledge of informal lay care giving is crude indeed, but it *is* sufficient to conclude that mediating health structures are integral to culture itself. Judgments of their productivity must, therefore, take place at several levels of meaning and benefit. They are multipurpose resources often lacking the ordinary idea of purpose as consciousness of a goal. Parental care *may* be health care, but it is a complex of interactions and growth-promoting events that serve a very broad definition of health. In effect mediating structures are integral to culture and social life and as such possess advantages of service beyond the reach of artifactual forms of health service.

The cultural integrity of mediating structures defines their acceptability as part of an individual's or a group's identification with its culture. There is no discordance between a given mediating resource and its clients. Which mediating structures are used and how often depends on their availability. Most of us most of the time live with access to many, but rarely all, mediating structures. There is variation in mediating constellations through time and personal life stages. The synchronization of availability with needs is not always assured; indeed the alienation of youth and the isolation of elderly are testimony to lack of access to mediating resources. The utility of mediating structures is indeed most starkly demonstrated in their absence.

## Health Benefits of Pluralism

Mediating structures in health are pluralistic in form and function. This is evident in our heterogeneous society. The more pertinent observation is that pluralism establishes the role of mediating structures as the essential modality of service, particularly the service of protection. A multiplicity of cultural filters screen out or render impotent many of the demands made by mass society on individuals. Evidence of this resistance is plentiful in the instance of educational and social campaigns aimed at achieving public conformity to values and behavior that require voluntary compliance. The health establishment devotes considerable effort to increasing levels of compliance, "targeting" populations that are "hard-core" resisters. There is a vast behavioral science technology designed to penetrate the beliefs that thwart adoption of prescribed health behaviors. Perhaps the most dramatic example of successful resistance was the swine flu vaccine program of 1976. We are able to see, in this failure of public acceptance, the power of mediating structures as they assessed the validity of the problem (what was the risk of flu) and the efficacy of the solution (what was the risk of the vaccine).

The power of mediating structures in protection is by no means solely a process of avoiding or reducing inappropriate or unacceptable public demands of megastructures. There also is a more immediate and intimate effect: the control of iatrogenic effects consequent to seeking and using organized professional services. In Chapter 4 we cited the example of family control in the use of medical services by urban Gypsies. More ordinary examples of the role of mediating structures in controlling the counterproductivity of health services are seen in the advisory process of the lay referral system and in the health care shopping process. Variations in family interpretations of symptoms, triggering cues to seeking care, and perspectives on treatment options blunt the iatrogenic potential inherent in any service monolith. The megastructure is increasingly under pressure to particularize its services and to share information on risks as well as benefits. Clearly the health establishment has received strong encouragement to do so by groups both governmental (the Federal Trade Commission, the Office of Technology Assessment) and private (Ralph Nader's health research group). These agencies support effective lay decision making through information on health hazards, both environmental and therapeutic. But their most profound effect may be on legitimating skepticism and assertiveness as essential elements in lay protection in a massified, alienating, and commercialized society. This contribution to the empowerment of people, of course, nurtures the ability of mediating structures as resources that cannot be relied on to serve the interests of any health ideology as represented by purveyors of harm or purveyors of help. Paternalistic solutions in health promotion are subject to lay mediation as surely as are the more obviously hazardous aspects of medical care.

Perhaps the most powerful contribution of mediating structures to protection in health is their role in the disease-labeling process. The health care system establishes its policies, prerogatives, and programs on an agreed range of values, which constitute diagnostic and treatment categories. Although often wide latitude of clinical judgment is involved and in the case of some chronic conditions only arbitrary definitions are available, a reasonable consensus often forms and is adopted by the professions. This consensus may be shared by the public in some instances, as in the case of diabetes, while for other conditions (or symptom clusters) it may not, as in the case of mild hypertension or some forms of mental disease. Disease is, ultimately, culturally defined deviance. Criteria are derived from various clinical belief structures, but it is the wider culture that determines the tolerable limits of a deviance category. These are not static determinations. Negotiations are always in process with regard to what constitutes substantial deviance warranting purposeful intervention by the individual, family, or competent professional. The norm for this process has always ranged from somewhat to substantially discordant. The lay community usually seems reluctant to widen the definition of deviance, sensing an erosion of personal control resulting in risk of pain, loss of status, stigmatization, institutionalization, or a succession of iatrogenic effects. Lay people are committed to a negative diagnostic finding. Health professionals, on the other hand, are socially chartered to find and treat disease in both active and incipient states. Their purpose demands methods that are both sensitive (widest possible production) and specific (most definitively determined). Here the commitment is to arrive at a positive diagnosis and to carry through a treatment plan.

Mediating structures constitute the agencies that negotiate the lay terms of reference with regard to labeling. Their importance in this respect has grown more critical and more obvious as the pattern of disease has increasingly become one of chronic disease. Now the issue is not so much a matter of arguing the meaning of acute symptoms but of dealing with the *illness* implications of long-term chronic disease. The effects of labeling are often as disabling as the underlying clinical pathology. It is easy to appreciate the public intuition to avoid labeling and where possible to restrict the categories of behavior construed as deviant. Some health professionals view this situation as "denial" and urge efforts to help people accept their illness as an important step in therapy. The issue is a complex one with competing technical and ideological values. But it is clear that the social implications of illness are of vital interest to its victims and their mediating resources. As chronic diseases continue to dominate and aging itself is labeled a pathology, we can expect a sharpening resistance to both blaming the victim as the cause of her problem and blaming the victim for the consequences of resisting professional labeling.

## Political Effectiveness

Mediating structures in health constitute a political dimension of social life that establishes and protects the identity and growth of its members. But their political state is rarely politically affiliated with any consistent value system associated with American political philosophies. In effect they are both the process and the product of American democratic pluralism. They are by no means ignored, nor are their status and welfare beyond controversy. The cancellation of the 1978 White House conference on the family as a result of volatile differences with regard to the definition of family is clear testimony to that.

The perceived nonaligned status of mediating structures in health does not necessarily mean a neutral stance on their part on specific health issues. We see, for example, substantial interventions of the churches and coalitions of women's groups in policy on abortion. Members of mutual aid groups, by sharing personal experiences, identify problems associated with their welfare that demand solution in political action. This level of political interest speaks to another aspect of mediating structures as having a powerful identity with their respective constituencies. Mediating structures can be and often are politically active in pursuit of the interests of their immediate constituents, but it is this very condition of particularity that denies their reliability as contributors to a political hegemony in health. The power of mediating structures lies in their pervasiveness, in their particularity, and in their consequent ability to withstand effective political control. Mediating structures, on the other hand, should not be seen as parochial and purely self-interested. Some mediating structures do exercise their broader political interest through coalitions and networks.

## Response to Need

The service of mediating structures in health care can be characterized generally as pragmatic and self-generating. By and large escaping the value constraints of the established health bureaucracy, mediating structures appear in response to needs that do not require formal legitimating procedures that test the reality of need against objective, external criteria. No certification of need directs parents with regard to nurturing care of children; no assessment of systems failure precipitates the growth of healing ministries; and no experimental evidence of the benefits of mutual aid was used to promulgate this form of care. The genius of mediating resources in health is their pragmatism in responding to needs and preferences. For the most part, the technology involved in health promoting, protecting, and caring is learned endogenously through intergenerational socialization, shared peer experience, and participation in particularizing cultural institutions. Formal indoctrination in health skills remains peripheral in comparison with these informal sources of learning.

The implications of the natural genesis of mediating structures in health clearly are most powerful with regard to the benefits of virtually universal availability and accessibility. But there is a qualitative point to be made as well. One could look at mediating structures in health as a vast array of empirical tests going on over long periods. They are not committed to any single value system, scientific or otherwise, and in effect enjoy liberation from most inhibiting factors external to the beliefs and experience of the participants. There is an opportunity (often no choice) to approach a problem or master resources in ways not necessarily concordant with methods used by the professional care system. This has not infrequently led to health care innovations of substantial consequences, which are later adopted by health professionals. Examples of these innovations have been noted many times in this book.

Two other, closely linked qualitative aspects of mediating structures deserve special emphasis as we consider public policies affecting them. By definition the process of nonprofessional health care is rooted in participation of the beneficiary. The help comes in large part from within the individual or group and is thus empowering and developmental. These are important psychological and social residuals that participation contributes to the giver-recipient well beyond the satisfaction of an immediate need. The effectiveness of mediating structures in health can be validly summarized only in indicators of public competence in health and confidence in that competence.

With participation comes direct accountability. The result is the ultimate in market sensitivity. Participation diminishes substantially or ceases altogether when satisfaction with the process or results drops away. This is most obvious in mutual aid groups, as noted earlier, but it is equally true in relation to self-care, the use of family and friendship support, healing ministries, and lay volunteering. Criteria for accountability (service quality) fit the circumstances of participation in care and therefore embody judgments pertinent to an *interactive* situation. This contrasts with consumer judgments of professional services, where criteria are unidimensional, that is, effects of the service *on* the person, not *with* the person. When the outcome of help is substantially a product of the participant's input, satisfaction is determined in good part on the basis of judgments of enhanced personal integrity, self-worth, and accrued personal power in health control. They are developmental criteria seldom used in evaluating professional health services.

## Benefits for Traditional Care

Mediating structures stabilize the professional care system or at the very least make it possible for services to keep up with demand. Even a modest drop in the amount of care offered by mediating structures could have a serious effect on the ability of professional resources to meet needs. On the other hand, an equally modest rise in the contribution of nonprofessional care resources might easily force substantial reductions in demand for professional care services. Although the precise relationship of mediating structures to professional resources with comparable health care interests is unknown (a matter we shall return to), it is logical that where present and potential service overlap, we must assume the dominant role of lay resources in deploying professional services.

## THE VULNERABILITY OF MEDIATING
## STRUCTURES IN HEALTH

As is true of other aspects of culture and social life, mediating structures in health naturally metamorphose. They reflect and at the same time define the state of the human arts in observation, communication, and caring. Health customs and beliefs, though often appearing stable and resistant to change, probably owe this reputation more to their resilience than to their rigidity. Increasing interaction among various cultural subsets and their mutual exposure to the official medical culture accelerate the transition of beliefs and practices to new configurations. Although some lay health practices are prescribed by religious laws and are therefore somewhat protected from change, studies of lay health practices in the United States show them to be substantially secular, influenced by general aspects of culture and social position.

The relative openness of culturally based health practices contributes to their vitality and relevance as they are passed from one generation to the next and as they disperse among social groups. The informal peer review process of pragmatic tests helps, but by no means guarantees, protection of lay health practice from abuse and exploitation. There are myriad examples of market intrusions in the form of products or procedures offered as solutions to specific health problems. The lay health resource is also subject to epidemics of health fads that move swiftly through the population and disappear. These intrusions are sometimes commercially motivated (for example, cancer cure products) and sometimes professionally induced (such as avoidance of cholesterol). Despite the proliferation of pressure points on lay health practices, however, there is no evidence that those practices on the whole have deteriorated. Indeed, there are strong suggestions that they are, for example, a factor in the reduction of mortality from heart disease. There appears to be no justification for the view held by some health professionals that the American people are a mindless mass of masochists bent on self-destruction through self-diagnosis and self-treatment.

Mediating structures are vulnerable to such criticism but appear unaffected by it, if we can judge by the continuing surge of interest in self-care, mutual aid, and other forms of lay health initiatives. Nevertheless, this perspective on self-harm could have a chilling effect on support for public policies designed to strengthen existing mediating structures or to encourage new lay health care opportunities. Even more insidious in this respect is the potential for this fear to grow to the point of counterproductive paternalism. School health education curricula, for example, could be kept at their present generally benign level with little emphasis on taking charge of one's body, demystifying health, and deprofessionalizing primary health care. Presumably, such a paternalistic approach to child health education also would avoid teaching skills in posing health problems and dealing with the political realities of health and health care on the grounds that a little knowledge of such matters would be more dangerous than no knowledge of them at all.

Another de facto constraint to which mediating structures in health are vulnerable is, ironically, a product of their newly recognized status by health professionals eager to assist in improving them. Here the danger lies in the conversion of effectively integrated social behaviors to self-consciously ministered health activities. This process of medicalization can result in a form of lay professionalism, which *may* achieve (there is no assurance) some technical benefits but at the same time may erode or replace aspects of the lay caring process that have several levels of value well beyond the immediate technical benefit. The health care nuance in parental care, the synergistic effects of mutual aid groups, and the peer insights of the lay volunteer in a suicide control center are the fragile essence of those agencies of caring. The teaching of professionally oriented procedures without sensitivity to and regard for the implicit values of mediating structures in *their* personal meaning could have multiple negative effects. In addition to the loss or downgrading of endogenous methods of care, there is a potential for increased lay dependency on professional judgments of right and wrong and a corresponding heightening of lay concern for their failure to perform as expected by the health authority. We must remind ourselves that professional services are supplementary to mediating structures and that mediating structures can and do contribute to the efficacy of the professional care system. Erosion of their integrity would be at high cost to the entire health care enterprise.

De facto developments are the most pervasive and probably the most hazardous influences on the continuing viability of mediating structures in health. In contrast, de jure factors relevant to the status of mediating structures are, at the moment, more intimidating than influential. Yet there are on the books laws and regulations regarding health care that could pose very real problems for the expanding health roles of mediating structures. Before proceeding to several examples, it is important to stress that the several state laws governing the *practice* of health care, particularly, medical practice acts, were first promulgated several decades ago and that, despite frequent amendments, they remain essentially intact. These laws reflect the values, needs, and expectations of a society quite different from the present one. In the years since the practice laws were established, there have been major changes in disease patterns requiring more caring than curing, a rise in average education level, and development of home care technology. Along with these changes, alternatives to traditional medical care have flourished, as evidenced in the public interest in self-care, home birth, the healing ministries, and mutual aid groups. Legislation embodied in the medical practice acts has not kept pace with these social changes. The result is a serious discordance of these acts with the actual practice of health care in the community.[2]

Common sense would seem to discount any real concern about a literal application of professional medical practice acts in constraint of popular and customary health activities (like home remedies). Nonetheless, the laws are in place and have occasionally been brought to bear. There is, in effect, room for arbitrary and selective enforcement of the medical practice acts. This has been demonstrated in several diverse instances of prosecution of lay persons doing abortion counseling or suggesting yogurt treatment for vaginal infection or even of city officials for fluoridating a town's water supply.[3] Although such suits were not successful, they can be an intimidating portent of a broader sweep. At least a partial remedy in the case of state medical practice acts would be to narrow their application to practitioners who provide services for a fee.

Mediating structures are also vulnerable at the hands of a variety of statutes and administrative directives that restrict access of lay persons to technical and professional support services. An example is the public health laboratory. Despite evidence of the efficacy of home throat cultures, for example, the public ordinarily cannot avail itself of this resource.[4] From every reasonable perspective of need, competence, and civil establishment, it is in the public's interest to have access to laboratory facilities to achieve wider public protection. Clearly this would entail adjustments of administrative procedures, but the cost-benefit yield would more than compensate.

As seen in the home birth movement, professional resistance can coalesce with binding professional codes to exert the force of law. The threat of losing hospital staff privileges can be an effective deterrent to physicians who would otherwise be available and willing to deliver babies at home. In the name of protecting the public interest, professions can stand on their codes of ethics, codes that have not been subject to lay review, much less input. In effect, the health care role of mediating structures that provide any form of health care has no legal standing. As the breadth of mediating resources expands into established professional jurisdictions of service, we can expect to see increased litigation and the prospect of precedent-setting decisions. Given the political volatility of some of the issues that will surely be raised (as in the case of women's free clinics), a most useful strategy for protecting the contribution of mediating structures would be legislative, in the first instance supported by the participation of lay representatives on boards of control and enforcement.

## IMPLICATIONS FOR HEALTH POLICY

To speak about health policies in the United States is problematical. It is more accurate to speak about health programs where a general policy is obscure if it exists at all. Nevertheless, one can discern some common values that underlie statements of program goals and methods to achieve them. There is no doubt that, despite allowances for consumer participation in some planning activities, the major commitment of health programs is to a professional construction of health and health intervention. This view holds that the history of health and health care is synonymous with the history of medicine and professional medical care: the health care system refers to the professional resource. Health care workers are professionals. In planning, we distinguish easily between providers and consumers. Health care costs are defined as expenditures for professional services and related technical accessories.

The construction of health and health care based on professional values and criteria is not an easy one to penetrate. It is the bedrock assumption on which the health care autocracy has been built.

Debate on how to modify the system is lively and varied, but all pro-posals fall into the context of the professional solution. Mendelsohn and his colleagues use the example of national health insurance proposals:

> Regardless of the particular scheme advocated, those with a vested interest in "health delivery" win. Physicians and their institutions (hospitals, the drug industry, insurance companies), having narrowed the definition of health services to the services they control and provide, now stand to maxi-mize their control by taxing every American.[5]

How, then, can (or indeed should) the case for mediating structures be made? The answer, we believe, lies in the larger domain of social change itself, where political realities place practical constraints on programs regardless of the enthusiasm of their architects. In the case of professional health services, the political reality is becoming clearer. As one economist observed with regard to health care, "If you don't gain much by a little more, you won't lose much with a little less." The shrinking relative productivity of professional care is only one dimension of this reality. Competition from other social needs is exemplified in recent union contracts calling for increases in take-home pay rather than increases in health and other fringe benefits. Perhaps most significant are shifts in (or reassertion of) social values that seek greater personal empowerment and wider personal options.

As endogenous phenomena, mediating structures in health are not a political coalition in the usual sense of providing a focused challenge to existing health programs. There is no evidence of an overall move-ment that collides with established programs and demands their withdrawal. For example, the three in-depth discussions of specific mediating structures' health activities revealed three very different relationships with, and effects on, the professional resource. In the home birth movement, there is a clear jurisdictional conflict, which has spawned considerable publicity and even some lawsuits. Religious healing, on the other hand, has coexisted quite compatibly with professional medical care and has avoided any suggestion of competi-tion with it. The example of rape crisis centers lies somewhere between. Although these volunteer agencies have taken an advocacy role on behalf of patients, many have met with considerable success in changing institutional practices and even generated innovations in medical treatment. The pressure for change within the established health system comes from the broadening of the social perspective on health care, which places professional services as one among many alternatives in health care. Corollary to this are a growing sense of precision in the mix of health care resources, including the personal resource, and, inevitably, the replacement of the professional mystique with respect for technical competence.

It is the secularization of health care that constitutes the medium for change within the professional system. This is most evident in examples of the doctor-patient relationship, which is transforming itself into an economic or bureaucratic model (provider-consumer) as health care becomes a more complex, interdependent service system. Lay access to health information and technology and to critiques of professional services contributes further to the erosion of the medical monolith, the conceptual protective shell of the medical monopoly.

The strain of transition from medical monotheism to health care pluralism is certain to show in the form of actions to slow or deflect the recognition, maintenance, and purposeful nurturance of mediating health resources. We noted how vulnerable mediating structures are to the power of the incumbent health care ideology and system. And there is more than a hint that the professional system will exercise its privilege through the law or through expanding its own venue of responsibility. Some of the resultant stress may be helpful in sorting out, in balancing resources, and in making ample time for revisions in our commitments to training, deploying, and financing professional resources. The influence of mediating structures on professional health services will continue to be largely evolutionary as episodes of crisis (cost burdens) or as effective inventions (mutual aid) occur. While in this sense nature may take its course, it may also take its toll.

We can grasp now the constructive potential of the alliance of social and professional health resources and can implement strategies of preservation, adjustment, and development that can be immediately productive.

## Preserving Existing Structures

Preservation of existing mediating resources is clearly the first priority. In formulating health policies, we must first be conscious of their potential harmful effects on individuals and the collective.

Policies must consider the social ecology of the problems they address and in effect develop an impact statement analogous to that required for legislation that may have environmental implications. The importance of this strategy for the preservation of mediating structures is illustrated in legislative proposals for a national meals-on-wheels program. Although it is not strictly viewed as a health program, the health implications of meals-on-wheels are obvious and profound. We cite meals-on-wheels as an instructive example because it is the only relevant contemporary policy development that has undergone careful study from the standpoint of its impact on mediating structures. In his review of the legislative history of meals-on-wheels and current proposals, Michael Balzano identified factors in legislation to expand and strengthen meals-on-wheels programs that could negatively affect essential elements of private, nonprofit programs already in operation.[6] These grass-roots programs are started largely by volunteers, many of whom share the social and cultural values of their clients. The volunteer represents a vital link to the outside world as a neighbor and friend. Most of these programs are small and privately sponsored by local social groups. Some receive subsidies through the United Way as well as a very small amount of federal money. Most of the programs appear to be highly regarded and in fact contribute to the cohesion of neighborhood and community.

A new federal initiative to broaden access to meals-on-wheels is contained in the 1978 amendments to the Older Americans Act (Part C of Title III). Ostensibly favoring as a first priority the strengthening of existing meals-on-wheels programs, the proposed legislation and subsequent regulations would in fact drive existing programs out of the federal support system or cause their discontinuance altogether. Balzano identified four specific requirements that could precipitate a negative effect on existing volunteer programs: that nutrition education be provided to program recipients (when the recipients prefer *not* to change their dietary habits); that there be a project council to advise the program director (which could conflict with existing advisory resources); that there be a minimum size for qualifying a meals-on-wheels program, mandatory staff training, and a full-time project director (which would wipe out programs serving under 100 meals or force expansion regardless of effects on quality and efficiency); and that meals conform to universal nutritional specifications (which may conflict with local preferences).[7]

The pattern of decision making with regard to federal legislation on meals-on-wheels demonstrates little effort to gain representative information on existing programs and to assess the experiences of longstanding, apparently successful programs. Clearly, equity of access to meals-on-wheels must be expanded to meet a growing need. It would seem especially prudent, therefore, that legislation support extant local resources, learn from them as well as instruct them, and encourage the extension of services in forms that achieve the greatest acceptability. The latter point is ultimately the crucial one. The protective value of mediating structures can be most contributory through its harmony with client values and its ability to particularize (customize) its services.

From the example of the analysis of meals-on-wheels legislation, we can sense the importance of some form of regular review of health and health-related legislation from the standpoint of its implications for mediating structures.

We recognize the limitations of any administrative solution and its potential for cooptation and misrepresentation. But it is necessary at the same time to give visibility to the crucial role of mediating structures and their contribution to policy options. Furthermore, advocacy in the interest of mediating structures must achieve some consistency among issues and not be selectively applied to those that have historically attracted attention through their implications for mediating structures, such as day care, independent living for the handicapped, and foster homes.

## Restructuring Health Care

Adjustments in the sensitivity of professional health care givers to the role of mediating structures must accompany political action. Powerful ideological commitments held by health professionals form barriers to any change that may reduce their power or their venue of practice. To crowd awareness of mediating structures into their perceptual field can be expected to meet lack of interest or, at the most extreme, resistance. Health professionals are under seige: specialization is limiting responsibilities; a system of services imposes regulations; and national health insurance is at the center of political debate. A consideration of the role of mediating structures in health would further separate the professionals from their professionalism by expanding the scale of health services and locating professional activity in a broad context. This would reveal the professional activity as a technical one, critical but specific. Further, the idea of a lay health resource may be unwelcome as one that would blur distinctions between consumers and providers and cause a breakdown in the discipline associated with these roles. The education and work settings of most health professionals have the effect of desensitization with regard to the functions of mediating structures. If mediating structures are considered at all, it is usually in terms of their pathogenic contributions (families as a source of disease) or as residual resources (dealing with minor problems of no interest to the professional).

None of this is meant to suggest that no leverage points are available for changing such views among health professionals. Leverage points do exist, for example, in medical and nursing education, in altering existing work settings, and in developing innovations in delivering and paying for health services that are responsive to mediating structures.

Curricula in community medicine and nursing often combine academic and practical experience in learning how health care can be most effectively delivered to communities. Here is an opportunity to explore the other side of the health care system, the "community's medicine." This curriculum would explore the following kind of questions. What are common self-care practices? How do families provide care in acute and chronic disease? What are the distinctions in the health care roles of extended families and friends? Who participates in mutual aid groups, and how do these groups function? What is the role of the church in health care? Are lay volunteers a factor in community health care? Gaining a perspective on mediating structures could serve to place professional intervention in its most productive context. This should also reduce the professionals' cynicism resulting from anxiety associated with their view of themselves as solely responsible for health care in an unhelpful, even hostile, environment. In effect, mediating structures may come to be seen as a support system for the health professional as well as for clients.

Strategies to adjust professional perspectives on mediating structures are also available in existing institutional settings. As we noted earlier, lay volunteers are both affected by and affect professional staff. Familiarity in these situations usually breeds respect for the interdependence of their roles. But for the most part, health professionals work in relative isolation from mediating structures at such an obvious level. More subtle interactions of professionals with mediating resources abound but are often less visible. The most obvious and ordinary contact is with the families of patients. Too frequently they are seen as interfering with care when the objective is to seek their cooperation with professional judgments in contrast with seeking their active participation in decision making. Indeed, the caring institutions—hospitals, nursing homes, even day care centers—do not usually encourage the presence and involvement of family and friends as sources of protection (advocacy) or support (love). Yet these are contributions to care that can be provided best by mediating resources.

Approaches to increasing the role of mediating structures in institutional care settings might consider ways of raising the credibility of mediating structures as valuable in concrete cases. In the long term, however, we must address the larger issue of the institutional environment itself as essentially hostile to the impact of mediating structures on patient care. Where people are reduced to disease labels, organs, or room numbers, staff members are not likely to value their patients' mediating resources. Professionals whose work is heavily routinized, hierarchical, and stressful (physically and psychologically) are often subject to burnout, described as "emotional exhaustion in which the professional person no longer has any positive feelings, sympathy, or respect for patients or clients."[8]

Other aspects of the institutional environment, which perhaps appear more benign, nonetheless contribute to the institutionalization and disabling of patients and the atrophy of their mediating resources. Routines organized for the efficient control of the curing process may often have damaging consequences for the healing and caring process. For example, the separation of mothers and infants after birth is efficient from the standpoint of hospital routine but may lead to social iatrogenic consequences for the family. We might now borrow from the example of the hospital infections committee, set up to investigate and control nosocomial infections, and establish a similar device to evaluate and control routine impediments to the normal functioning of mediating structures, particularly the patient and family.

Adjustments to existing modes of training and work setting notwithstanding, it is also necessary to consider adjustments in the financing and organization of health services from the point of view of mediating structures. There is an often expressed view that the level of use of mediating health resources, especially self-care for minor illnesses and injuries, is related to the way people pay for professional health services. This view holds that if third-party payment is involved, there will be a tendency for people to "abuse" the system by seeking professional help for many problems they would otherwise treat themselves. Thus approaches to insurance mechanisms are proposed that would eliminate alleged abuses through high deductibles or requirements for coinsurance or both. Available evidence from countries with full prepaid coverage and those with fragmentary coverage suggests, however, that the level of self-care practices is about the same. The mere presence or even character of insurance is not substantiated as an important determinant of self-care. Furthermore, the case for using insurance as a lever for increasing self-care is flawed by its reliance on a definition of "minor illness and injury"—a definition that downgrades lay judgments in favor of professional criteria. This could lead to abuses of the client with little or no accountability of the professional provider.

A more productive approach to nurturing the self-care option would be one that provides the professional system with incentives to share health care responsibility with its clients. The health maintenance organization (HMO) is such a model of health care delivery. Support of its clients' independence is in the clear interest of the HMO.[9] The clients' control of self in personal care and in managing the contribution of professional care are goals compatible with the HMO ideology as well as with administrative reality. Economic, social, and health benefits to provider and consumer are both overlapping and unique. There is, however, no automatic assurance that HMOs will take special advantage of the opportunities for strengthening the lay health resource. Indeed, their current struggle to achieve adequate membership may postpone attention to investments in self-care education. Furthermore, the form of the HMO is a key factor in influencing its educational potential. Independent practice associations (IPAs), affiliations of private practitioners scattered throughout a community, seem to be a less hospitable organizational plan for purposes of self-care education (or at least, less accountable) than the closed-panel HMO, where services are provided in a group practice setting under one roof. We urge, therefore, that support grants and regulations governing HMO development reflect an educational priority and, in the IPA form, make additional provisions for educational services through a common resource accessible to all IPA members, regardless of their choice of care provider.

### Encouraging Self-Care

In considering strategies for developing mediating structures in health, we are confined to a frame of reference that emphasizes nurturing of these natural social resources and precludes attempts to manipulate or restructure in the interests of a better fit with professional services. We are guided by the principle caveat, *primum non nocere,* to ensure that the integrity of the structures remains as an expression of individual and community preference and style. Developmental changes in the form and function of mediating structures will result as pragmatic experience dictates.

There are two strategies that meet the criterion of being developmental without necessarily being manipulative: public education and networking. Neither, of course, is immune from abuse, but they are the generic tools of social development and as such represent the best opportunity to move with the social will and to be responsive to it.

The mediating structure that is most accessible and appropriate to education is the individual self-provider of health care. Self-care education for adults has proliferated since the early 1970s.[10] These programs vary by sponsor, clients, content, methods, evaluation, and funding. They share a general goal, however: to help people take more effective control in health. More specific objectives may include learning about the body, personal and environmental causes of ill health, protection strategies, care for minor illnesses and injuries, chronic disease management, self-medication, and safe and effective use of professional health resources. Health and health care are demystified, and health technology is transferred to lay use. The expected result is a shift in the locus of control in health from professional to lay person.[11]

Development of self-care education is an innovation that holds promise of broad appeal to diverse populations with varying beliefs about health and preferences about health care. The base of access to self-care education must be broadened to include groups at particularly high risk of disease and iatrogenic effects of professional care: minorities, the poor, and the elderly. Educational methods also require revisions that would allow people to determine their own learning needs and assert their own learning styles. The educational approach itself must be exemplary of the objective to empower people.

To achieve wider distribution and access will require concentrated financial support for programs to reduce or eliminate the barrier of fees and the barrier of sponsorship now heavily concentrated in the health care sector. Neighborhood libraries, for example, can provide unique benefits of access as well as an environment that could avoid allegiance to any one dominant health care ideology. For rural populations, the county extension office of the U.S. Department of Agriculture may be an appropriate sponsor. Voluntary associations, social clubs, women's groups, and service organizations offer a special opportunity to particularize self-care education in the interests of their constituencies.

Technical information, medications, and technology are nearly universal components of effective competence in medical self-care. Effective access to these resources is a major factor in the continuing development of the lay health care role.

The sharp rise in the number and variety of print media resources is impressive, and these are soon to be complemented by software for home-controlled television viewing. We can anticipate innovations in educational communication that will tie together the now disparate elements of home health records, health risk appraisal, and diagnostic and treatment protocols, in effect providing a sophisticated and highly particularized home-based information system to support lay health decision making. The benefits of these developments are clear, and it is essential that both equity of access and relevance to diverse social groups be ensured. Commercial enterprise must be supplemented by publicly supported research, development, and distribution beyond the mainstream middle-class market. This calls for an evaluation of existing strategies and priorities of federal investments in health education and a reallocation of effort toward designing home-based health information *systems* available to all the people.

The availability of nonprescribed medications (over-the-counter preparations) has been a traditional and useful resource in lay health care. Although they have often been deemed merely palliative, recent Food and Drug Administration decisions to release more active ingredients to direct public access require consideration of their curative benefits as well. In either case, the role of over-the-counter preparations is an essential one both for health benefits to the user and for the viability of the professional system. To the latter point, an economist reminds us that even relatively small shifts away from the present level of self-medication toward professional care would require immense expansion of professional resources.[12]

Increasing access to safe and effective active ingredients through over-the-counter products is in the public interest. We agree with one experienced Food and Drug Administration review panel member that "the entire list of prescription drugs . . . be scrutinized in the light of Section 503(b) 1 [of the Federal Food, Drug, and Cosmetic Act, 21 USC] for further scientifically proven agents that could be made more easily available to the public."[13] At the same time it is necessary to strengthen public information about the utility of over-the-counter drugs as a legitimate component of the health care system and the specific utility (benefits, limitations) of any given medication at point of sale. Similarly, the health professions need information about the rational substitutability of over-the-counter for prescribed medication.[14] Health education of public and professional is clearly the most important way to normalize the contribution of nonprescribed drugs in the total care system. Vastly more attention must be given by the Bureau of Health Education (Center for Disease Control) and the Office of Health Information and Health Promotion to this aspect of medical self-care.

Closely aligned to medication as a central component in lay self-care is the more recent availability of home health care technology. Since 1975 we have seen a wide range of diagnostic, monitoring, and treatment technology added to the traditional household standbys of thermometer, hot water bottle, and elastic bandage. Adaptations for lay use of devices previously limited to professional use and the addition of new ones developed expressly for lay use are finding ready public acceptance. In the diagnostic category, for example, new technology includes home throat cultures, diabetic self-monitoring, bowel cancer screening, detection of urinary tract infections, home blood pressure monitoring, and pregnancy testing.[15]

Government review of medical technology for home use provides some assurance of its effective use under prescribed circumstances. There remains a need, however, to simplify technology further and at the same time to educate consumers in its proper application. Market competition may help eliminate cumbersome design, but the potential for consumer error inherent in the use of some technology will require that educational materials be available in school health education programs, at the point of sale (packaged patient inserts, pharmacies), in medical care facilities, and in media advertising.

Several self-diagnostic technologies, such as home throat culturing, require the assistance of a competent laboratory. Unfortunately, the availability of such laboratory resources is restricted to patients whose physicians or health care plans will voluntarily cooperate or to those who have access to, and can pay for, private laboratory service. Public health laboratories traditionally limit their services to physicians, clinics and hospitals, and public health departments. Service to private individuals is usually not available. This situation is both inequitable and inappropriate and should be corrected through revision of state statutes governing public health laboratory operations.

Self-care education of children needs special attention. The educational environment in American schools is in many ways hostile to an educational strategy that encourages problem posing in contradistinction to an exclusive emphasis on problem solving.[16] Further, there is a commitment to mainstream beliefs about health and the appropriate health care jurisdictions of lay people and health professionals. The history of school health education shows how it has avoided clarifying the notion of ownership of the body and useful skills in self-management, such as diagnosis and treatment. And perhaps its greatest deficiency is health education's adherence to the view that one's health record is an autobiography rather than a social history with powerful political and economic determinants.[17]

We were unable to find any report of a comprehensive self-care school health education program. Substantial demonstrations are under way, however, that emphasize key components. One outstanding example is a six-year demonstration program in an elementary school in Hartford, Connecticut, where primary medical and dental services involve children in the care process as participants as well as recipients. Children assist the health professionals in self-care and peer care in a way that reveals the causal factors, nature, and implications of a given pathology and the rationale underlying treatment options. Mystery is replaced by understanding, and the children sense the legitimacy and satisfaction in gaining control over health care.[18]

A departure from traditional school health education will require the precedents of diverse and widespread demonstrations. Federal interest in school health education must be freed of pedagogical inheritance that commits it to the support of educational methods designed to modify behavior without strengthening the essential ability of children to define problems and to maintain the locus of health control within themselves. A review of school health policies and procedures from the standpoint of their nurturance of the individual as an effective mediating resource should be given high priority.

A second approach to enhancing the development of mediating structures is networking. There is a substantial and growing body of theoretical literature[19] and practical experience[20] on networking as a community development strategy. The concept is self-expressive of both its intent and its method. Simply stated, networking is putting community resources in touch with each other as a way of promoting their synergistic benefit to the community as a whole. When applied to mediating structures, the process confronts the obvious fact that we are not dealing with a homogeneous group of resources either in their structure or their dispersion. How can one conceptualize a process of collating such diverse resources as individuals, families, friendship networks, mutual aid groups, voluntary associations, and religious groups? The answer is that they are already linked in various direct and indirect ways, but they do not see themselves as a network with common interests in service and growth in effectiveness. The goal of intervention is to create community self-awareness of the referral resource and to maximize opportunities for mutual support among its components.

Networking is not an independent enterprise. It is a method of mobilizing mediating resources in the satisfaction of community health needs. In Chapter 1 we suggested that these support resources have four general functions: emotional support, identity provision and maintenance, providing information and influencing judgment and perception, and facilitating tasks. In many respects these contributions cannot be feasibly substituted for by official or professional structures. Too often, however, they are either ignored or taken for granted in community health planning. In either case an opportunity is lost to benefit from them and to strengthen their individual and collective abilities to respond to health needs. Planning policy must involve a purposeful initiative to network the mediating health resource. Further, the concept of mediating structure imposes its own matrix of functions within the general categories of expressive and instrumental functions. We are forced, however, to work with a mélange of evidence of mediating structures as they contribute to health and health care without benefit of a coherent data base.

The problem before us is to develop validated, reliable information on how mediating structures naturally coalesce, as a guide to health planning strategies. Conservation of the professional resources in health, we argue, is contingent on the productivity of mediating structures (in ways that are only partially clear). Given the social and economic limits, as well as the productive limits, of professional resources, a strategy that raises even modestly the efficiency of the pervasive mediating resource has much to recommend it. Neither vast new investments in professional resources[21] nor excessive reliance on paternalistic health controls[22] seems to be as feasible or purposeful as an organized strategy for identifying mediating resources, increasing their knowledge of their mutual interests, and facilitating concerted action based on their unique capabilities. This is not an administrative device to parcel out the community health problem for various mediating resources to work on. On the contrary, it is an attempt to learn how these resources now relate to the health concern and to learn from them how the official and professional structures can facilitate their joint effort.

## RESEARCH ON MEDIATING STRUCTURES FOR POLICY DEVELOPMENT

Throughout this book we have stressed the fragmentary and often marginal state of our knowledge of mediating structures generally and as they specifically relate to health. Part of the problem is the diversity of mediating structures, their forms, and their purposes.

Demographers, anthropologists, epidemiologists, sociologists, psychologists, economists, and organizational analysts, among others, have contributed much to our understanding of the entities that constitute mediating structures.

To plan for increments in the effective yield of mediating resources requires a profile of those resources in terms sufficient to (1) identify their relative values and (2) assess the circumstances and costs associated with interventions to accelerate their benefits. Circumstances will have to be particularized and costs examined in political as well as fiscal frames. Given the pluralistic and endogenous nature of mediating structures, the research goal here is to achieve *not* a uniform, centralized policy of development but rather a uniform method of accounting for and evaluating mediating resources.

Available methods of observing and quantifying health functions, designed primarily for the measurement of professional productivity in health care, cannot appropriately be applied to the study of the health care functions of mediating structures. Research on self-care practices, for example, has had to rely on secondary professionally constructed observations such as questionnaires and interviews. These are inadequate methods on several counts. First, it is clear that the definition of what constitutes health behavior in both expressive and instrumental categories must be derived from the mediating structure itself, be it an individual or a mutual aid group. Although some secondary observations may report high reliability coefficients, the question of validity remains. There is no basis for an assumption that professional and lay criteria for defining health behaviors are identical or even comparable. Although some behavioral items may be common to both, they are probably fewer than one might expect. Temperature taking is an example. There are many possible interpretations of this. Perhaps what is meant is the use of a thermometer. Parents asked whether they took their child's temperature may say no when in fact they "took the temperature" by placing a hand on the child's forehead. Expressive health behavior, particularly providing psychological support, may be as benign as the companionship of a friend. More structured situations of care may involve criteria of behavior equally at variance with professional judgments. And it may be even more difficult to correlate the clinical aspect of healing ministries with established allopathic criteria.

There is the problem of knowing what constitutes a valid observation and the companion problem of measuring its occurrence. Qualitative analytic methods may be helpful here, particularly "grounded theory" approaches.[23] The power of phenomenological methods resides in their particularity, not their generalizability beyond a given study population. Explanations of changes in the status of the public's health could benefit from a more carefully "grounded" appraisal of lay health behavior, promotive, preventive, and restorative. Epidemiological and descriptive social research on the relation of life-style to risk of disease is sufficiently encouraging to make more sophisticated qualitative analyses a high priority. Many of the findings raise as many questions as they appear to answer. There is, of course, the question of the validity of observation. But there is also the issue of explaining the mechanisms underlying the associations of behavior with health status. An example is the work of Berkman and Syme cited earlier. These authors demonstrate a dose-response relation between mortality experience (all causes) and an individual's friendship structure. What it is about friendships that makes the difference in mortality experience is a matter of speculation, however. Is it an expressive (supportive) contribution, or is it instrumental activities (care giving), or is it both? For obvious reasons, it is not feasible to take what is usually the next research step after epidemiological identification of potentially complicit factors, that is, a matched-control, double-blind clinical trial. On the other hand, qualitative methods are ideally suited to the tasks of isolating the relevant factors.

Mediating structures accumulate approaches to care giving from many sources, uninhibited by commitments to methods prescribed by the dominant allopathic professional health care system. They are an eclectic cluster of beliefs and practices subject to continuous pragmatic test. Improvisations and innovations come out of personal experience. Many of these ideas and practices find their way into the mainstream of public life. Others do not. It is not at all clear how effective health care innovations are now diffused from the often parochial confines of families and mutual aid groups, for example, to the wider community. What are the characteristics of a lay health practice that will predict its diffusion? What is the diffusion process as it applies to the various categories of mediating structures? How might the diffusion process be facilitated while avoiding the potential hazard of megastructural controls (such as quality control, regulating public access)? Research on these and related questions can make a substantial contribution to strengthening the credibility of mediating structures by harvesting the universal benefits of this highly pluralistic social resource of health care.

Ultimately, the purpose of our observations of mediating resources is to apply these data to local situations and to adapt our professional resources accordingly. The sector of national health policy that responds to this planning model would achieve a relevance, flexibility, and economy unavailable to present planning strategies based on clinical needs assessment in the absence of preference characteristics, formula ratios of manpower to population, fixed problem solutions, and an assumption that lay health resources represent no resource at all or equal units of incompetence. We cannot conceive of a rapid departure from the present planning ethic but rather an exploration of qualitative methods that can generate data that can help us account for the in-kind contributions of mediating resources and reveal the basis for their further development and supplementation with professional resources. Our view is that the key to an effective national health policy is its commitment to empowering local resources with responsibility for planning. The Health Services Agency (HSA) is a useful model in this respect, but its operating venue, with few exceptions, has been limited to professional or official agencies and resources. There is virtually no accounting for mediating resources. The need is for valid qualitative analyses and planning mechanisms to link qualitative data on mediating resources with the data base for allocating professional resources.

The federal establishment in health research has only occasionally explored the possibilities of mediating structures.[24] An overwhelming commitment to research confined within parameters of the professional system has left little interest and even fewer resources available to support a *coherent* program of research on mediating structures in health and health care. Without a concept of mediating structures in health as a rational and significant social resource, it is not likely that we shall see much more than scattered research with little or no chance of filling the need for a consistent body of knowledge. The map of mediating resources would remain partial and lack dimension.

Some will argue that the general lack of interest on the part of government and universities in mediating structures is assurance of protection from eventual regulating incursion or damage from being overstudied. We believe that while concern is justified, a lack of credible data on a substantial portion of our overall health care system places mediating structures in even greater jeopardy.

## A FUTURE PERSPECTIVE

Twenty million joggers, an estimated 10 to 12 million people participating in mutual aid groups, and approximately 3,500 current titles in the lay health literature provide concrete evidence of America's awakened health consciousness. A 1979 national probability survey found that 70 percent of those interviewed were more concerned about their health than they were the previous year and that 60 percent do not take good health for granted.[25]

Some observers have cautioned that the current surge of interest in health is one symptom of a narcissistic culture.[26] Others, taking note of the growing interest in holistic health and alternative (non-allopathic) care systems have labeled these events anti-intellectual, antigovernment, antisocial preoccupation with self, social cynicism, paranoia about computers (massification), or just a passing fad. One thing is clear: health has become a broadly based social activity well beyond the traditional domain of professional resources. Definitions of health and how to achieve it derive from a multiplicity of social values and beliefs. Similarly, the concept of care giving appears to have abandoned confinement to a strictly medical model. What is the impetus for these developments, and what might be their effect on our national interest in health? We posit that the following factors and forces are among the most important contributors to the resurgence of mediating structures' activities in health and the public interest in them.

### Caring for the Chronically Ill

Over the past forty years or so, there has been a substantial shift in the pattern of disease from approximately 30 percent of all diseases being chronic to the present 80 percent. This has had two effects important for mediating structures. The first is the inability of medical care delivery to adjust adequately to this rapid change, leaving much of the system dysfunctional for meeting the special needs of the chronically ill, particularly that of help with the psychological dimensions of long-term illness and effective management skills. The public has learned to limit its expectation of medical expertise to providing initial treatment regimens and help at times of exacerbation of chronic problems. A second consequence of the morbidity shift, compounded by the limitations of medical assistance, has been the public discovery that other resources, including families, friends, and mutual aid groups, are useful in providing support and ideas with regard to day-to-day management. Many lay people who believed they have little to offer in terms of *cure,* now find they can contribute a good deal to *care.*

## Holistic Health

As a corollary we can observe an increase in the availability and appeal of alternative health care strategies, many of which are self-administered or appropriate for lay groups. Meditation, relaxation, and biofeedback techniques are examples. Along with this has come a resurgence of interest in religious healing ministries. Eastern health and healing practices have been appealing options as well. An over-arching perspective on the holism of health and health care has emerged with a central commitment to the views that health is more than the absence of disease; the body, mind, and spirit are interactive and complementary; and the health of individuals is linked to the social and physical environment. Holistic health is an eclectic concept, and its practice is highly diverse.[27] As a result its appeal is wide. Severe critiques by the allopathic establishment notwithstanding,[28] holism is having some obvious impact on the system (American Holistic Medical Association) and, perhaps, more subtle effects in challenging medical monotheism. In this respect it is interesting to note federal cosponsorship of a national forum on holistic health and public policy.[29]

## Beyond Medicine

A growing research literature has clarified and documented the role of factors other than medical on health status. Economic, behavioral, social, cultural, and environmental sources of stress are clearly not

influenced by medical care. Effective interactions therefore lie beyond medicine's capability. As a result, its social charter for service
in prevention is undergoing an invisible but palpable revision. The
public is turning to more relevant remedies through environmental
protection control of safety hazards, humanizing the work place,
housing and employment initiatives, education, and changes in
life-style. Federal health policy proposals reflect these realities regarding strategies for prevention.[30] Expectations of improvement in
the nation's health status have shifted to a focus on individuals,
families, and larger social collectives, although specific strategies
lack precision. Individuals, for example, are often blamed for the
state of their health, when it is clear that larger environmental con-
siderations are involved. It is a curious irony that mediating resources
must now provide protection from some of the very strategies that
seek to empower people, such as behavior modification.[31]

### Altering the Doctor-Patient Relationship

Medicine as an alternative to mediating structures in health has been
subject to considerable devaluation in terms of productivity, safety,
and exclusivity. Recent studies in Britain and the United States have
demonstrated a relatively modest contribution of medical care to
health and to the control of disease.[32] Public awareness of this point
is difficult to assess. Indicators of demand for physician services, for
example, have not fluctuated very much since 1972, suggesting little
or no reduction in the public's perception of the general usefulness
of medical care. On the other hand, information on the safety of
professional health services is widely disseminated in the public
press[33] as well as in scholarly literature.[34] But of greater impact is
the direct experience of patients whose contact with medical care
has caused additional clinical problems. Apparently there is a ready
audience for popular magazine articles and books on how to protect
oneself from the hazards of medical care.

The exclusivity of medicine as embodying tightly circumscribed
roles for its practitioners has been breached. Functions previously
the exclusive domain of physicians are now distributed among
others, such as physician associates and nurse practitioners. Further,
as health care becomes increasingly bureaucratized, the role of practitioners becomes secularized. The doctor-patient relationship is now

a provider-consumer relationship. It is an economic model with consequent changes in attitudes and expectations. The cost of care is becoming nearly as important a public concern as the question of quality. In effect, professional medical care has entered the marketplace where shoppers may (and do) assert their options both among professional choices and between those choices and nonprofessional resources. While this has always been possible, the secularization of medicine as a profession certainly must enhance the social acceptability of the process.

### Public Empowerment

Finally, there is an impression of a rising tide of populism, symbolized by California's famous (or infamous) Proposition 13. Some see in that political act (and a spate of copies elsewhere) a signal that Americans feel that they have lost control over the important institutions of their lives and will not tolerate further erosion of their personal control over them. They want more decentralization, more accountability, and more personal involvement in decision making as solutions to perceived widespread inadequacies in, and abuses by, both public and private megastructures. This has stimulated a powerful public interest in collective action to improve the quality of life and equity in its achievement. We agree with Berger and Neuhaus that "what first appears as contradiction, then, is the sum of equally justified aspirations. The public policy goal is to address human needs without exacerbating the reasons for animus against the welfare state."[35]

Public response to the medical megastructure is our case in point. Although there has been no dramatic consumer revolt, there are ample signs of disenchantment with medicine's promised benefits, however inappropriate or exaggerated such promises may be. Disappointments have been expressed about costs, yield, access, and quality. Especially there are concerns that the integral role of the individual has been neglected or even excluded from the health care process. The term "dehumanized" is often applied. Medical care often disables self-determining behavior, self-healing abilities, self-control in care, and growth of the individual in self-actualizing ways. Medical care appears to be more draining than fulfilling, more usurp-tive of power than empowering. But having acknowledged these resentments and disappointments, the public experience seems not to abandon or withdraw support for professional health services. The response is to be more cautious in the use of these services, yes, and at the same time to consider or reconsider mediating care resources. This represents greater precision in the public's perception of the contribution of medical care and, as a corollary, greater awareness of the legitimate potential of self and other mediating health resources and of the need to activate them more consciously. It is not an either/or situation but a desire to maximize the potential of both sources of help.

The emergence of mediating structures in health is a consequence of wider changes in society. There is no basis for defining what is happening as a movement in the classic sense. Nonetheless, we can see perhaps more clearly now than in the recent past the existence of an authentic health service resource profoundly social in character and function, highly pluralistic, and growing in its self-awareness. The intent of this book is to draw attention to the present and potential contributions of mediating structures and to argue for an approach to policy in the public sector that would enhance and protect them. They are clearly in the public interest as the public has defined it in their current vitality and creativity. But mediating structures serve also to enhance and protect the public interest in the continuing availability of professional care. We are hopeful that public policy, sensitive to the vital private role of people in their health and health care, can arrive at collective actions that accept people as resources as well as recipients.

## REFERENCES

1. Pope Pius XI, "The Concept of Subsidiarity," *Quadragesimo Anno* (1931).
2. Lori B. Andrews and Lowell S. Levin, "Self-Care and the Law," *Social Policy* 9, no. 4 (January-February 1979): 44–49.
3. [3]Ibid., p. 44.
4. [4]Harvey P. Katz and Robert R. Claney, "Accuracy of a Home Throat Culture Program: A Study of Parent Participation in Health Care," *Pediatrics* 53, no. 5 (May 1974): 687–91.
5. Robert Mendelson, John McKnight, and Ivan Illich, "National Health Insurance and the People's Health," *Clinical Pediatrics* 12, no. 6 (June 1973): 324.

6.  Michael P. Balzano, *Federalizing Meals-on-Wheels: Private Sector Loss or Gain?* (Washington, D.C.: American Enterprise Institute. 1979).

7.  Ibid., pp. 31-32.

8.  Christina Maslach, "The Burn-out Syndrome and Patient Care," in Charles A. Garfield, ed., *Stress and Survival: The Emotional Realities of Life-Threatening Illness,* (St. Louis: C.V. Mosby, 1979), p. 113.

9.  Patricia Mullen, Kathleen Kukowski, and Sarah Mazelis, "Health Education in Health Maintenance Organizations," in Peter Lazes, ed., *The Handbook of Health Education,* pp. 53-76.

10. Keith W. Sehnert and Joseph T. Nocerino, "Course Guide for the Activated Patient: A Consumer Oriented Program in Preventive Medicine," Georgetown University School of Medicine, Department of Community Medicine and International Health, 1974, mimeo.

11. Robert M. Silten and Lowell S. Levin, "Self-Care Education," in Peter M. Lazes, ed., *The Handbook of Health Education* (Germantown, Md.: Aspen Systems, 1979), pp. 201-21.

12. Simon Rottenberg, "Self-Medication: The Economic Perspective," *Self-Medication: The New Era, A Symposium,* (Washington, D.C.: Proprietary Association 1980), p. 30.

13. E. William Rosenberg, "Self-Medication and Science: A Partnership," *Self-Medication: The New Era, A Symposium,* (Washington, D.C.: Proprietary Association, March 31, 1980), p. 9.

14. An example of a useful resource for pharmacists and physicians: *Handbook of Nonprescribed Drugs,* 6th ed. (Washington, D.C.: American Pharmaceutical Association, 1979).

15. For a review of newly available diagnostic techniques for lay use, see David S. Sobel, "Self-Diagnostic Tests," *Medical Self-Care* (Summer 1980): 14-17.

16. Paolo Freire, *Pedagogy of the Oppressed* (New York: Seabury Press, 1974).

17. Lowell S. Levin, "Self-Empowering School Health Education," *Proceedings of the Conference on Discovering Health Power* (New Haven, Conn.: Teacher Center, April 28, 1979).

18. Judy Lewis, "Toward Comprehensive Child Health Care: A School-Based Delivery Model," paper presented at the American Public Health Association Annual Meeting, Washington, D.C., 1977 (mimeo.).

19. H. Turk, "Interorganizational Networks in Urban Society: Initial Perspectives and Comparative Research," *American Sociological Review,* Vol. 35 (1970), pp. 1-19.

20. Seymour B. Sarason et al., *Human Services and Resource Networks* (San Francisco: Jossey Bass, 1977).

21. Fuchs, *Who Shall Live?*

22.  Daniel I. Wikler, "Persuasion and Coercion for Health: Ethical Issues in Government Efforts to Change Life-Styles," *Milbank Memorial Fund Quarterly/Health and Society* 56, no. 3 (Summer 1978): 303–38.

23.  Anselm Strauss and Barney Glaser, *The Discovery of Grounded Theory: Strategies for Qualitative Research* (Chicago: Aldine, 1967); Glaser, *Theoretical Sensitivity.*

24.  National Center for Health Services Research, *Research Proceedings: Consumer Self-Care in Health,* U.S. Department of Health, Education and Welfare, No. (HRA) 72-3181, August 1977; Bureau of Health Education, *Self-Care,* United States Department of Health, Education and Welfare, Center for Disease Control, Atlanta, Georgia.

25.  Yankelovich, Skelly, and White, Inc., *The General Mills American Family Report, 1978-1979: Family Health in an Era of Stress* (Minneapolis: General Mills, 1979).

26.  Christopher Lasch, *The Culture of Narcissism,* (New York: Norton, 1979).

27.  David S. Sobel, ed., *Ways of Health: Holistic Approaches to Ancient and Contemporary Medicine* (New York: Harcourt Brace Jovanovich, 1979).

28.  Arnold S. Relman, "Holistic Medicine," *New England Journal of Medicine* 300, no. 6 (February 8, 1979): 312-31.

29.  East-West Academy of Healing Arts Forum on Holistic Health: A Public Policy, Washington, D.C., April 1978.

30.  U.S. Department of Health, Education and Welfare, Public Health Service, Office of the Assistant Secretary for Health, *Health: United States, 1978,* "Determinants of Health," pp. 201-29.

31.  Carl I. Cohen and Ellen J. Cohen, "Health Education: Panacea, Pernicious or Pointless," *New England Journal of Medicine,* vol. 299 (September 1978), pp. 718-20.

32.  Thomas McKeown, *The Role of Medicine;* John B. McKinlay and Sonja M. McKinlay, "The Questionable Contribution of Medical Measures."

33.  An example of press coverage of the negative aspects of medical care is a series appearing in the *New York Times,* January 27-30, 1976.

34.  P.E. Sartwell, "Iatrogenic Disease: An Epidemiological Perspective," *International Journal of Health Services,* vol. 4, no. 1 (1974), pp. 89-90; Nikola Schipkowensky. *Psychotherapy versus Iatrogeny: A Confrontation for Physicians* (Detroit: Wayne State University Press, 1972).

35.  Peter L. Berger and Richard John Neuhaus. *To Empower People: The Role of Mediating Structures in Public Policy* (Washington, D.C.: American Enterprise Institute, 1977), p. 2.

# INDEX

267

# ABOUT THE AUTHORS

**Lowell S. Levin** is Professor of Public Health at the Yale University School of Medicine, Department of Epidemiology and Public Health. His scholarly and political interests in public health have moved increasingly toward the contribution and potential of nonprofessional health resources. As senior author of *Self-Care: Lay Initiatives in Health,* together with numerous articles and lectures, he has added substantially to our understanding of the lay health resource, particularly its requirements for research. His current studies address the process and problems of shifting control in health care from professionals to lay people.

**Ellen L. Idler** is currently a student in the Ph.D. program in sociology at Yale University. She has worked as a volunteer for several women's health organizations. Her published work is concerned with the theoretical differences between professional and nonprofessional definitions of health and illness. Ms. Idler's special interest is in the religious, historical, and traditional sources of health knowledge.